Respiratory Problems in Primary Care

RCGP Curriculum for
General Practice Series

Respiratory Problems in Primary Care

A guide for new GPs

Edited by
Rachel Booker,
Monica Fletcher,
Simon Gregory and
Stephen Holmes

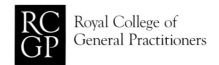

Royal College of
General Practitioners

The Royal College of General Practitioners was founded in 1952 with this object:

'To encourage, foster and maintain the highest possible standards in general practice and for that purpose to take or join with others in taking steps consistent with the charitable nature of that object which may assist towards the same.'

Among its responsibilities under its Royal Charter the College is entitled to:

'Diffuse information on all matters affecting general practice and issue such publications as may assist the object of the College.'

British Library Cataloguing-in-Publication Data
A catalogue record for this book is available from the British Library

© Royal College of General Practitioners 2009
Published by the Royal College of General Practitioners 2009
14 Princes Gate, Hyde Park, London SW7 1PU

Disclaimer
This publication is intended for the use of medical practitioners in the UK and not for patients. The authors, editors and publisher have taken care to ensure that the information contained in this book is correct to the best of their knowledge, at the time of publication. Whilst efforts have been made to ensure the accuracy of the information presented, particularly that related to the prescription of drugs, the authors, editors and publisher cannot accept liability for information that is subsequently shown to be wrong. Readers are advised to check that the information, especially that related to drug usage, complies with information contained in the *British National Formulary*, or equivalent, or manufacturers' datasheets, and that it complies with the latest legislation and standards of practice.

Designed and typeset at the Typographic Design Unit
Printed by Hobbs the Printers Ltd
Indexed by Carol Ball

ISBN: 978-0-85084-320-0

Contents

Contributors

Rachel Booker BSc RGN DN Cert HV is an independent specialist respiratory nurse and freelance writer, formerly COPD and Spirometry Module Leader at Education for Health, Warwick. She is also author of *Vital COPD, Vital Lung Function*, and co-author of *Chronic Obstructive Pulmonary Disease in Primary Care*, now in its third edition. In 2007 the Queen's Nursing Institute awarded her the Queen Elizabeth the Queen Mother's Award for Outstanding Service.

David Fishwick FRCP (London) FRCP (Glasgow) AFOM is a Reader in Respiratory Medicine and honorary Consultant Respiratory Physician at the University of Sheffield and Royal Hallamshire Hospital, Sheffield. As his main clinical and research interests relate to breathing at work, he is also co-Director of the Centre for Workplace Health and the Chief Medical Officer at the Health and Safety Laboratory.

Monica Fletcher BSc (Hons) MSc PGCE is a primary care nurse by background and is currently the Chief Executive of Education for Health, an international medical education charity that trains health professionals in a range of long-term conditions. She is Chair of the Primary Care Group of the European Respiratory Society (ERS) and a council member of the European Lung Foundation (ELF). She is a member of the Executive Committee of the BTS/SIGN Asthma Guidelines Group. She is an active member of the American Thoracic Society (ATS) Nursing Assembly and is a member of the ATS International Lung Health Committee.

Simon Gregory FRCGP FHEA is a GP at King Edward Road Surgery in Northampton and is General Practice Postgraduate Dean for the East Midlands Healthcare Workforce Deanery. He is also a nationally elected member of the RCGP Council, a Vice-Chair of the Committee of General Practice Education Directors (COGPED) and the Editor-in-Chief of *General Practice Update*. In addition to medical education his main clinical interest is respiratory disease in primary care, focusing in particular on chronic obstructive pulmonary disease (COPD).

Roswyn Hakesley-Brown CBE BA MPhil FRSH RN RM RNT Cert Ed is an independent consultant in healthcare education. She is currently working on the smoking cessation curriculum for nurses and midwives for the Department of Health. She is also closely involved in the integration of refugee healthcare professionals into the NHS workforce and is Chair of the Patients Association.

Yvonne Henderson MCSP is a respiratory physiotherapist with a particular interest in breathlessness management and pulmonary rehabilitation. She is a clinical lecturer and researcher at Education for Health in Warwick.

Stephen Holmes FRCGP DRCOG is a GP in Shepton Mallet, Somerset, and is education lead for the General Practice Airways Group (GPIAG). A former Chair of GPIAG, he is involved with the RCGP on the Professional Development Board, having been Chair of the Severn Faculty, and is currently a member of the RCGP Council. Steve is also an Associate Director in Medical Education at the Severn Deanery. He is also a member of the British Thoracic Society (BTS)/Scottish Intercollegiate Guidelines Network (SIGN) 'Living Asthma Guideline' executive and the British Thoracic Society Education Committee, as well as of the Asthma UK Healthcare Forum executive.

Carol Min MRCP (London) is a specialist registrar in respiratory medicine at Heatherwood and Wexham Park Foundation Trust, and is currently training in the Oxford Deanery. Her main interest is lung cancer.

Aziz Sheikh FRCP FRCGP DCH DRCOG is Professor of Primary Care Research and Development at the University of Edinburgh, where he is Head of the Allergy and Respiratory Research Group in the Division of Community Health Sciences'. He is an Honorary Consultant Allergist in NHS Lothian and Research Adviser to Education for Health.

Iain Small FRCGP is a general practitioner in Peterhead, Aberdeenshire. He is the Chair of the GPIAG, clinical lead for the Grampian Managed Clinical Network for COPD, and an honorary lecturer in the Department of Primary Care at the University of Aberdeen. He is a trainer for Education for Health, and sits on the Professional Advisory Committee for Asthma UK (Scotland). He was for many years Chair of the Scottish Paediatric Asthma Group, and sat on Quality Improvement Scotland's Children's Asthma Standards Group.

Samantha Walker PhD RGN is Director of Education and Research at Education for Health in Warwick and Honorary Senior Lecturer in the Division of Community Health Sciences at the University of Edinburgh. She is a nationally elected member of the British Society for Allergy and Clinical Immunology Council, chairs its Primary Care Group and is an active member of the Standards of Care Committee. She is also research lead for the GPIAG.

John Wiggins FRCP **(London)** FRCP **(Edinburgh)** is Consultant Physician at Heatherwood and Wexham Park Foundation Trust. He is a member of the Council
of the British Thoracic Society and Chair of its Mesothelioma Working Party.
His interests include lung cancer, tuberculosis and interstitial lung disease.

Foreword

Serious respiratory diseases kill one in four people in the UK and are the most common reason for general practice consultations, accounting for 25 per cent of a GP's workload and 30 per cent of all hospital admissions.

It is vital that, as GPs, we understand the principles of diagnosis and treatment for common conditions, and that we have the competence and confidence to know when and when not to prescribe.

Added to this, health promotion through smoking cessation and lifestyle advice is becoming increasingly important in primary care – as is the need to fully involve patients in the management of their respiratory problems.

The publication of this excellent book is therefore very timely. As well as covering the breadth of respiratory infections, their common causes and presentations, it brings together guidelines and resources in an easy-to-reference way that all GPs should find useful.

My thanks to the authors (Rachel Booker, David Fishwick, Monica Fletcher, Simon Gregory, Roswyn Hakesley-Brown, Yvonne Henderson, Stephen Holmes, Carol Min, Aziz Sheikh, Iain Small, Samantha Walker and John Wiggins) for all their hard work in bringing together so much information in such a clear and accessible format.

I'm sure that this will become a must-have publication for GPs and trainee GPs everywhere.

Prof. Steve Field
Chairman of Council, Royal College of General Practitioners
January 2009

Acknowledgements

The editors would like to thank the chapter authors for working so hard and Helen Farrelly of the RCGP for her patience and support during the long gestation of this book.

We would also like to thank colleagues at Education for Health and in the General Practice Airways Group for their support and encouragement to produce a book aimed at those training for and working in careers as general practitioners.

Abbreviations

AAT	alpha 1 antitrypsin levels
ABG	arterial blood gas
ACE	angiotensin-converting enzyme
ACQ	Asthma Control Questionnaire
ACT	Asthma Control Test
AECOPD	acute exacerbation of COPD
AIIA	acute irritant-induced asthma
APMS	Alternative Provider Medical Services
AR	allergic rhinitis
ATS	American Thoracic Society
b.d.	twice daily
BDP	beclometasone dipropionate
BMI	body mass index
BOHRF	British Occupational Health Research Foundation
BTS	British Thoracic Society
CAP	community-acquired pneumonia
CF	cystic fibrosis
CHART	continuous hyperfractionated accelerated radiotherapy
CO_2	carbon dioxide
COGPED	Committee of General Practice Education Directors
COPD	chronic obstructive pulmonary disease
CRP	C-reactive protein
CT	computerised tomogram (computerised axial tomography scanning)
CXR	chest X-ray/radiograph
DOT	directly observed treatment
DPI	dry powder inhaler
DWP	Department for Work and Pensions
EAA	extrinsic allergic alveolitis
ECG	electrocardiogram
ELF	European Lung Foundation
ENT	ear, nose and throat/otorhinolaryngology
ERS	European Respiratory Society
ETS	environmental tobacco smoke
FBC	full blood count
FDG	fluorodeoxyglucose
FEV_1	forced expiratory volume in one second

FiO$_2$	fraction of inspired oxygen
FTND	Fagerström Test for Nicotine Dependence
FVC	forced vital capacity
GMS	General Medical Services
GOR	gastro-oesophageal reflux
GORDS	Group of Occupational Respiratory Disease Specialists
GPIAG	General Practice Airways Group
GPStR	general practice specialty registrar (formerly known as GP registrar)
GPwSI	General Practitioner with a Special Interest
HOOF	Home Oxygen Order Form
HRCT	high-resolution CT
HSE	Health and Safety Executive
ICS	inhaled corticosteroid
IgE	immunoglobulin-E
IgG	immunoglobulin-G
IM	intramuscular
IV	intravenous
JVP	jugular venous pressure
kPa	kilopascals
LABA	long-acting beta-agonist
LFT	liver function test
LRTI	lower respiratory tract infection
LTOT	long-term oxygen therapy
LTRAs	leukotriene receptor antagonists
LVF	left ventricular failure
LVSD	left ventricular systolic dysfunction
MDI	metered-dose inhaler
MDT	multidisciplinary team
MRC	Medical Research Council
MRI	magnetic resonance imaging
nGMS	new General Medical Services contract
NICE	National Institute for Health and Clinical Excellence
NNT	number needed to treat
NOTT	Nocturnal Oxygen Therapy Trial
NRT	nicotine replacement therapy
NSAID	non-steroidal anti-inflammatory drug
NSCLC	non-small-cell lung cancer
NSF	National Service Framework
O$_2$	oxygen
OA	occupational asthma

OPRA	Occupational Physicians Reporting Activity
OTC	over-the-counter medicine
PAF	platelet-activating factor
PAHs	polycyclic aromatic hydrocarbons
PaO_2	partial pressure of oxygen in arterial blood
PBC	Practice-Based Commissioning
PCO	Primary Care Organisation
PCP	*Pneumocystis carinii* pneumonia
PE	pulmonary embolism
PEF	peak flow
PEFR	peak expiratory flow rate
PET	positron emission tomography
pMDI	pressurised metered dose inhaler
PMS	Personal Medical Services
p.o.	by mouth
PRN	as needed
PTHrP	parathyroid hormone-related peptide
QOF	Quality and Outcomes Framework
RAAS	renin angiotensin aldosterone system
RAD	reactive airway disease
RADS	reactive airways dysfunction syndrome
RCP	Royal College of Physicians
RCT	randomised controlled trial
RIDDOR	Reporting of Injuries, Diseases and Dangerous Occurrences Regulations
RSV	respiratory syncytial virus
SABA	short-acting beta-agonist
SaO_2	arterial blood oxygen saturation
SER	significant event review
SIADH	syndrome of inappropriate anti-diuretic hormone secretion
SIGN	Scottish Intercollegiate Guidelines Network
SCLC	small-cell lung cancer
SMART	single maintenance and reliever therapy
SpO_2	capillary/peripheral blood oxygen saturation
SVC	superior vena cava
SVCO	superior vena cava obstruction
SWORD	Surveillance of Work-Related and Occupational Respiratory Disease
TB	tuberculosis
t.d.s.	three times daily

THOR	The Health and Occupation Reporting Network
URTI	upper respiratory tract infection
VDGF	vapours, dusts, gases and fumes
VQ	ventilation–perfusion scan
VTA	ventral tegmental segment
WHO	World Health Organization

The burden of respiratory disease

1

Monica Fletcher

Chapter aims

This chapter seeks to explore the burden of respiratory disease to society and to the individual. We will consider the prevalence of respiratory conditions, their cost and their impact.

Learning outcomes

▷ To understand the current population trends in the prevalence of respiratory conditions (community orientation).
▷ To appreciate the impact respiratory conditions have on individual patients and their families, society, the NHS and primary care (contextual aspect and holistic approach).
▷ To understand the central role of primary care in managing respiratory conditions, in particular asthma and chronic obstructive pulmonary disease (COPD) (contextual aspect).
▷ To appreciate the relevance of other primary care health professionals in the delivery of care.
▷ To understand the importance of person-centred care in the delivery of respiratory care (person-centred care).

Initial self-assessment

1 ▷ For an average general practitioner (GP) list of 2000 patients how many patients would you expect to be on the disease register with the following conditions:
   a. asthma?
   b. COPD?

2 ▷ List the elements of care that you feel a practice should demonstrate if it is to provide a high standard of respiratory care.

3 ▷ Consider the role of a GP with a Special Interest (GPwSI) in respiratory medicine. If there is one in your locality, what services does he or she offer and what are the advantages and disadvantages of this model of care? If there is no such service in your locality, what factors would you consider in deciding whether to commission such a service?

The size of the problem

There are over 30 respiratory diseases in the UK, affecting both children and adults. However, only the most common of these are covered in this book.

Over 8 million people in the UK suffer from respiratory problems and the prevalence of both respiratory and allergic conditions is increasing.[1,2]

Respiratory diseases have a major impact on both morbidity and mortality, and shamefully the UK has one of the highest death rates from these conditions in Europe.[3]

One in five people in the UK die from a serious respiratory disease, accounting for more deaths per year than those occurring from ischaemic heart disease.[1] Respiratory cancers account for almost 30 per cent of the deaths. Of these almost 120,000 deaths, 59,105 occur in females and 58,351 in men. Women are now four times as likely to die from respiratory disease as from breast cancer.

The human suffering is extensive and respiratory disease costs the UK over £6.5 billion per annum, of which £3.06 billion are NHS costs. Only one tenth of this expenditure is accounted for by hospital inpatient admissions, making this very much a primary care issue.[1,4-6] Additionally in 1999/2000 there were over 28 million working days lost due to respiratory illness, at a cost of over £2 billion.[1]

Key points

▶ There are over 30 respiratory diseases in the UK.
▶ Over 8 million people in the UK have respiratory diseases.
▶ The UK has one of the highest death rates from respiratory disease in the European Union.

Figure 1.1 ○ *Age-standardised death rates per 100,000 population from respiratory disease (2001)*

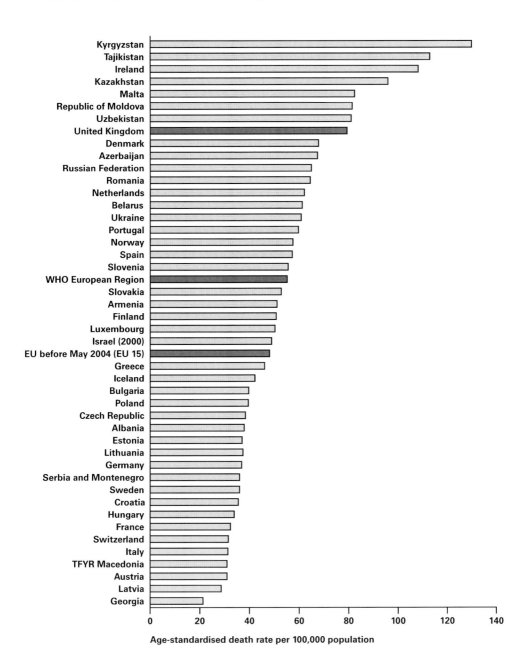

Age-standardised death rate per 100,000 population

3

Source: British Thoracic Society, p. 18.[1] Reproduced by kind permission.

Respiratory disease in primary care

Most respiratory conditions are appropriately managed in the primary care setting and the majority of patients are never seen by a respiratory consultant. Eighty-five per cent of asthma patients are managed totally by their GPs, and practice nurses.[7]

Respiratory illnesses, including upper and lower respiratory tract infections, are the most common reason why patients consult a GP. There are estimated to be 24 million primary care respiratory-related consultations each year,[1,8] which equates to about 3 per cent of all GP consultations.[9] When this figure is multiplied by the estimated unit cost of a GP consultation it gives a total cost of £501 million per year.[1] Many of these consultations are unscheduled appointments – 18 per cent of all GP emergency consultations are for a respiratory problem. In addition it has been estimated that 31 per cent of all adults and approximately 65 per cent of all children under 5 years will visit their GP at least once a year because of a respiratory condition, mainly acute infections, asthma and COPD[1] in adults.

Prescribing is also a big issue. In excess of 62 million prescriptions at a cost of £975.3 million were issued for the prevention and management of respiratory disease in 2004.[1]

Key points

▶ Most respiratory disease is managed in primary care.
▶ 85 per cent of asthma patients never see a hospital consultant.
▶ There are 24 million primary care respiratory-related consultations.
▶ 18 per cent of all GP emergency consultations are for a respiratory problem.
▶ 62 million prescriptions were issued in 2004.

Prevalence

The prevalence rates of respiratory diseases are increasing. The average GP with 2000 patients will have around 120 patients with asthma (see Chapter 4), whereas he or she will probably have 75–90 patients with COPD of whom 30 will be diagnosed as such (see Chapter 8). Lung cancer affects between 33,000 and 37,000 individuals per annum in the UK (new diagnoses), which accounts for 1 in 7 of all new cancer cases (see Chapter 9), and respiratory infections account for 25 per cent of a GP's workload and 30 per cent of all hospital admissions (see Chapter 11).

Figure 1.2 ○ *The relative burden of lung disease*

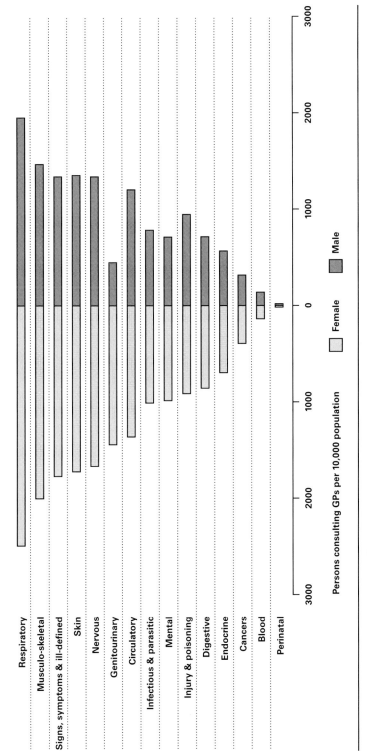

Persons consulting GPs per 10,000 population

Female | Male

Source: British Thoracic Society, p. 26.[1] Reproduced by kind permission.

Asthma is the major long-term respiratory disease in the UK and it is the most common chronic disease of childhood. Currently there are over 5.2 million people living with the condition of all ages and social backgrounds.[10] There is a wide range of severity of the disease but most people receive their treatment from their GP practice; however, over 70,000 hospital admissions are recorded annually for acute asthma.[10] Almost three quarters of these admissions are preventable. Despite great effort being made by primary care to improve the lives of people with asthma, many do continue to live with unacceptable levels of symptoms. The prevalence of active asthma reported in the Quality and Outcomes Framework (QOF) in 2007/8 was 5.7 per cent in England,[11] 5.4 per cent in Scotland,[12] 6.6 per cent in Wales[13] and 5.8 per cent in Northern Ireland.[14]

About 1.5 per cent of the population (900,000 people) are diagnosed with COPD. However, it is widely acknowledged that this is a gross underestimation and the true figure would be double this number.

A GP with an average list size of 2000 patients would have about 30 known cases of COPD, while a four partner, 8000-patient practice would have about 120; however, the real number could be as high as between 300 and 360. In areas of socioeconomic deprivation with high smoking rates the prevalence will be even higher. The prevalence of COPD reported in the QOF in 2007/8 was 1.5 per cent in England,[11] 1.8 per cent in Scotland,[12] 1.9 per cent in Wales[13] and 1.5 per cent in Northern Ireland.[14]

Over 30 per cent of the UK population suffer from allergic rhinitis and yet these conditions are often trivialised. However, the impact on quality of life is extensive.[15, 16]

Key points

▶ Over 5 million people are living with asthma.
▶ 70,000 people are still admitted into hospital per annum with acute asthma.
▶ 1.5 per cent (900,000 people) of the population are diagnosed with COPD.
▶ Over 30 per cent of the population suffer from allergic rhinitis.

Costs to the NHS

The cost to the health service of respiratory disease is more than any other disease and accounts for 2.8 million bed days a year. An estimated 1 million hospital admissions in 2004 were attributed to a respiratory cause.

Although there are fewer patients diagnosed with COPD than with asthma, considerably more people die from the disease than from asthma – about twenty-fold. In 2004 there were approximately 27,000 recorded deaths from COPD, compared with 1400 from asthma. What is worrying about the asthma deaths is that many are preventable and a third of these occur in people aged below 65 years. Confidential inquiries have shown suboptimal care and poor adherence to medication contribute to unnecessary deaths.[17-19]

Due to the number of hospitalisations and the length of stay, the annual cost of treating COPD is considerably higher. On average, patients admitted to hospital with COPD stay in hospital over three times longer (10.3 days) than patients admitted with asthma (3.6 days).[20] For an average Primary Care Organisation (PCO) with 250,000 patients the total cost for hospital admissions for both conditions is in excess of £1 million (see Table 1.1).

Table 1.1 ○ *Annual hospital admissions and related costs for asthma and COPD*

Hospital admissions	England (2000/1)		Typical PCO	
	Asthma	*COPD*	*Asthma*	*COPD*
Number of hospital admissions	52,706	101,713	220	425
Total number of inpatient bed days	169,717	1,014,632	709	4241
Cost per inpatient bed day	£229	£229	£229	£229
Total cost	£38.9m	£232.4m	£162,400	£971,200

Note: PCO estimates calculated for population of 250,000 relative to population of 50 million in England (mid-2000 estimate).

Source: National Respiratory Training Centre.[21] Reproduced by kind permission of Education for Health Warwick.

In a PCO of 250,000 there will be almost 16,000 consultations for respiratory disease per annum. This will cost about £2.5 million. Asthma and COPD in particular will account for a sizeable proportion of this. In a PCO of this size there will be over 21,000 patients being treated for asthma and 2500 for COPD.[21]

Key points

▶ Respiratory diseases cost the NHS more than any other disease.
▶ They account for 2.8 million bed days per year.
▶ Twenty-fold more people die of COPD per annum than asthma.

▶ In a PCO of 250,000 there will be almost 16,000 consultations per annum for respiratory disease, costing about £2.5 million.

Social inequalities

Deprivation and social inequalities cause a higher proportion of deaths in respiratory disease than any other condition. Forty-four per cent of all respiratory deaths are associated with class inequalities compared with 28 per cent from ischaemic heart disease. Furthermore men aged 20–64 years employed in unskilled manual occupations are around 14 times more likely to die from COPD and nine times more likely to die from tuberculosis than men employed in professional occupations. The standardised mortality ratio for respiratory conditions indicates a three-fold difference across all social classes.[1] There are however fewer regional differences in asthma mortality than in COPD.[21]

Raising the profile

Given the size of the problem and the workload placed on primary care it is astonishing that the management of respiratory disease does not attract a greater national NHS priority. This is possibly because primary care is already delivering most of the care.

Despite the immense burden placed on patients, the NHS and society as a whole, respiratory diseases are not deemed to be a national priority and are not one of the priority areas defined in the national strategy for health.[22] There has not been a National Service Framework (NSF) for respiratory conditions. An NSF would have represented a major drive to help address the gross inequalities in health status and provision of services. However, after considerable lobbying, a National Clinical Strategy has been developed for COPD that will be released later in 2009 and should go some way in addressing the inequities in care across the UK. The strategy will concentrate on prevention, diagnosis, management – both pharmacological and non-pharmacological – and end-of-life care. Other common respiratory conditions, including asthma and sleep apnoea, place a substantial burden on the health of the nation. It is essential that other chapters are commissioned to develop a uniform plan in the NHS for lung diseases, looking at their prevention and diagnosis and management.

In order to place a greater priority on respiratory disease in primary care, it will be helpful to establish the current impact on your practice, commissioning group and/or the primary care organisation. Tackling the manage-

---

Box 1.1 ○ *Questions for prioritising respiratory health*

▶ Does your PCO or Practice-Based Commissioning group know how many patients there are with respiratory disease, particularly the number of patients with COPD and asthma?

▶ Do these figures mirror the national figures?

▶ Do they reflect the local population as far as epidemiological and chronological determinants?

▶ How are these diseases identified by the practices?

▶ What are the local costs of treating patients with respiratory disease: inpatient, outpatient and primary care?

▶ What could be done differently?

---

ment of asthma and COPD in primary care should be viewed as high priority for primary healthcare teams.

The questions laid out in Box 1.1 could help in formulating a priority case for respiratory disease in your local area.

If the morbidity from and economic burden of respiratory disease are to be reduced, asthma and COPD must be addressed within Health Improvement and Modernisation Plans. It has been demonstrated that when this happens there can be significant improvements in practitioner behaviour, skills and expertise, and patient outcomes.[23]

Key points

▶ Despite the prevalence rates, respiratory disease is not deemed to be a national priority.
▶ A COPD NSF is planned for 2008.
▶ It is important to make a local needs assessment in order to prioritise in a local area.

The respiratory paradox

Respiratory diseases are very common conditions for which there are many effective pharmacological and non-pharmacological interventions available for use in general practice and the community. For diseases such as asthma, rhinitis and COPD there is a wide range of drug therapies and delivery systems to choose from. With advances in science there is a far greater understanding of the pathogenesis of respiratory diseases than previously, and as a result GPs are more knowledgeable about how to prevent asthma and COPD exacerbations. In addition there is a range of excellent local, national and international evidence-based guidelines to guide primary care professionals in their daily practice.

Remarkably, however, both morbidity and mortality statistics and other quality-of-life studies continue to show that patients experience a considerable burden of symptoms. There are many possible reasons for this paradox, which can be related to the healthcare system, health professional factors and patients.

▷ Is it that health professionals are failing to follow guidelines and recommended practice – competing priorities?
▷ Could it be that healthcare systems are constructed in a way that hinder the implementation of good care – perverse incentives?
▷ Is it that patients are just prepared to tolerate poor symptom control and simply choose not to follow recommended treatment regimens?

The answer could be a combination of these factors, but central to all of this is a lack of good partnership working and effective patient education, including the use of self-management and the limited use of personalised action plans.

Adherence

The best inhaler device is the one the patient uses! There are numerous studies highlighting the extent of non-adherence to drug treatment in patients living with long-term respiratory conditions. The resulting morbidity in respiratory patients imposes a huge burden not only on the patient but also on health resources.[24,25] It has been estimated that for severe asthma the savings produced by optimal disease control would be around 45 per cent of total medical costs.

As the burden of chronic disease rises, predicted to reach 56 per cent of the total burden of disease by 2020 globally,[26] poor control and adherence to therapy becomes a major source of increasing healthcare costs. If chronic disease management requires self-administration of treatment, adherence problems will be seen, no matter how severe the disease or how accessible the healthcare resources. In asthma, adherence rates for regular preventive therapy have been reported to be as low as 28 per cent.[27]

It is known that patients tend to be more satisfied with the care they receive when they are involved with the consultation,[28,29] that adherence to treatment regimens improves and there are better patient outcomes as a result.[30,31]

It is firmly acknowledged that the patient should be a partner in his or her care and not just a passive recipient.[32]

There is much that can be done to improve the way we interact with our patients in order to improve adherence, and educational resources are available to assist busy primary care practitioners.[33] Factors influencing adherence are listed in Table 1.2.

Table 1.2 ○ *Factors influencing adherence: some ideas for consideration*

	Possible causes	
Condition-related factors	GP lack of knowledge in treatment management and/or an inadequate understanding of the disease	Management of disease and treatment in conjunction with patients
	Short consultations	
Medication-related factors	Patient has poor understanding of the disease	Patient education beginning at the time of diagnosis and integrated into every step of asthma care
	Lack of training in improving adherence	Training in monitoring adherence for GPs
	Complex treatment regimens	Simplification of regimens
	Long duration of treatment	Education on use of medicines
	Frequent doses	Adaptation of prescribed medications
	Adverse effects of treatment	Continuous monitoring and reassessment of treatment
	Forgetfulness	
	Misunderstanding of instructions about medicines	
	Poor parental understanding of children's medications	
	Lack of perception of personal vulnerability to illness	

Continued over

Possible causes

Lack of information about
the prescribed daily
dosage/misconceptions
about the disease and
treatments

Persistent misunderstanding
about side effects

Systematic delivery of respiratory care in general practice

There are many essential key components required for the delivery of excellent primary care respiratory services.

Key elements of successful respiratory care

▷ Appropriate prevention programmes/strategies – smoking cessation.
▷ Requires a high index of suspicion.
▷ Timely and accurate diagnosis.
▷ Early referral when required.
▷ Carefully planned management – according to evidence-based guidelines.
▷ Patient education.
▷ Self-management plans.
▷ Integrated care pathways.
▷ Audit of practice.
▷ Suitably trained staff.

Prevention

Respiratory diseases have different causes and therefore require different preventive strategies. Smoking is a key factor in causing deaths from respiratory disease but there are also genetic, nutritional, poverty-related and environmental factors involved in most common conditions. GPs certainly have a key role in dissuading people from starting smoking and in helping them to quit. Looking at the current death rates from smoking-related diseases, slightly more women than men are dying. This reflects the growth in the number of women smoking in the 1950s and 1960s when it was a fashionable activity. It is of great concern that current statistics show that females are beginning to smoke heavily again.

Studies within primary care have shown that considerable improvements for patients with asthma can be achieved with: adherence to management guidelines;[34] specialist training for healthcare professionals;[35] and structured care with systematic review of medication, inhaler technique and compliance.[36]

Development of specialist roles in primary care

GPwSIs have been around for some time, particularly in respiratory care. The General Practice Airways Group (GPIAG) was established in 1987. Traditionally relationships between GPs and their respiratory colleagues in hospital have been good, and the strong links between primary and secondary care clinicians are generally valued, drawing on the resources of the two areas of care to the mutual advantage of patients and clinicians.[37] However, specialist respiratory roles have developed in primary care. The formalising of GPwSIs was introduced in *The NHS Plan* in 2000,[38] and these roles certainly challenge traditional models of specialist care. Although the numbers of respiratory GPwSIs was initially slow to develop, the GPIAG now suggests that they have increased substantially.[39]

The development of the specialist clinical roles in primary care has tended to focus on the GP role. However, the government is supportive of a multidisciplinary approach to developing clinicians with a specialist clinical interest, and nurses and other allied health professionals are being encouraged to develop these roles. Specialist respiratory care is not about titles but ensuring that patients have access to an appropriate health professional who can assess all of their needs and manage these effectively.

One of the key drivers for the development of nurses' role in respiratory care in general practice was the GP contract of 1990. This was when GPs were first remunerated for running mixed chronic disease management clinics and latterly, in 1993, when chronic disease management programmes for asthma replaced the concept of a clinic. GPs were encouraged to appoint suitably qualified and experienced nurses to undertake key roles in caring for people with chronic diseases and training programmes became available.[7]

Over the years roles have developed for nurses working with patients with respiratory disease. Some of these nurses work exclusively with patients who have respiratory disease, while others are generalists with a special

13

interest. All are fulfilling vital roles in improving the care of patients with respiratory disease as part of the primary healthcare team.

The roles that nurses are adopting in respiratory care vary but they all contribute to dealing with the burden of lung disease. Nurses need to be appropriately trained to take on the challenges of managing the complex care of patients with respiratory disease, particularly those with co-morbidities and complex health needs. A survey of lead practice asthma and COPD nurses, conducted in 2007, revealed that a large percentage had not received an appropriate level of postgraduate education to equip them fully with the skills and competences required.[7]

The GMS contract QOF was intended to incentivise GPs to diagnose and manage asthma and COPD more effectively. Evidence-based indicators are used to encourage and reward high-quality clinical care (see Chapter 13). To deliver such quality of care requires a team approach to the management of long-term conditions, and to involve patients in their own condition and thereby their own management.

References

1 • British Thoracic Society. *The Burden of Lung Disease: a statistical report from the British Thoracic Society* (2nd edn) London: BTS, 2006.

2 • British Lung Foundation. *Lost in Translation: bridging the communication gap in COPD* London: BLF, 2006.

3 • World Health Organization. *European Health for All Statistical Database*, 2001, www.who.dk/country/country.htm [accessed December 2008].

4 • Netten A, Curtis L. *Unit Costs of Health and Social Care* Canterbury: PSSRU, University of Kent, 2000.

5 • National Respiratory Training Centre. *Impact of Respiratory Conditions: a guide for primary care organisations* Warwick: NRTC, 2002.

6 • Department of Health. *Hospital Episode Statistics, England 2000–01* www.hesonline.nhs.uk [accessed December 2008].

7 • Upton J, Madoc-Sutton H, Sheikh A, *et al*. National survey on the roles and training of primary care respiratory nurses in the UK in 2006: are we making progress? *Primary Care Respiratory Journal* 2007; **16(5)**: 284–90.

8 • RCGP Birmingham Research Unit. *Weekly Returns Service Annual Report 2004*, 2005, www.rcgp.org.uk/PDF/bru_AnnualRep04.pdf [accessed December 2008].

9 • McCormack A, Fleming D, Charlton J. *Morbidity Statistics from General Practice, Fourth National Study 1991–1992* London: HMSO.

10 • National Asthma Campaign. Out in the open: a true picture of asthma in the UK today *Asthma Journal* 2001; **6(3)**: special supplement.

11 • The Health and Social Care Information Centre. *National Quality and Outcomes Framework Statistics for England 2007/08*, www.ic.nhs.uk/servicesnew/qof [accessed January 2009].

12 • Scottish Health Statistics. *Quality and Outcomes Framework*, www.isdscotland.org/isd/3305.html [accessed September 2008].

13 • NHS Wales. *Quality and Outcomes Framework*, www.wales.nhs.uk/sites3/page.cfm?orgid=480&pid=6063 [accessed September 2008].

14 • Department of Health Social Services and Public Safety. *Quality and Outcomes Framework*, www.dhsspsni.gov.uk/index/hss/gp_contracts/gp_contract_qof.htm [accessed September 2008].

15 • Juniper EF, Guyatt GH. Development and testing of a new measure of health status for clinical trials in rhinoconjunctivitis *Clinical and Experimental Allergy* 1990; **21**: 77–83.

16 • Walker S, Khan-Wasti S, Fletcher M, *et al*. Seasonal allergic rhinitis is associated with a detrimental impact on exam performance in UK teenagers: case-control study *Journal of Allergy and Clinical Immunology* 2007; **120(2)**: 381–7.

17 • British Thoracic Association. Deaths from asthma in two regions of England *British Medical Journal* 1982; **285**: 1251–5.

18 • Mohan G, Harrison B D, Badminton R M, *et al*. A confidential enquiry into deaths caused by asthma in an English health region: implications for general practice *British Journal of General Practice* 1996; **46**: 529–32.

19 • Bucknall C E, Slack R, Godley C C, *et al*. on behalf of SCIAD. Scottish Confidential Inquiry into Asthma Deaths (SCIAD), 1994–6 *Thorax* 1999; **54**: 978–84.

20 • Department of Health. *Hospital Episode Statistics 1999/2000*, 2001, www.dh.gov.uk/en/Publicationsandstatistics/Statistics/HospitalEpisodeStatistics/index.htm [accessed September 2008].

21 • National Respiratory Training Centre. *Impact of Respiratory Conditions: a guide for primary care organisations* Warwick: NRTC, 2002.

22 • Department of Health. *Saving Lives: our healthier nation* London: The Stationery Office, 1999.

23 • O'Reilly J F, Holt K, Houghton I, *et al*. Costs and benefits of a 3-step COPD health improvement programme in primary care based on a visiting spirometry service *Thorax* 2001; **56(Suppl III)**: 86.

24 • Gruffyd Jones K, Bell J, Ferenbach C, *et al*. Understanding patient perceptions of asthma: results of the asthma control and expectations (ACE) study *International Journal of Clinical Practice* 2002; **56(2)**: 89–93.

25 • Rabe K F, Vermeire P A, Soriano J B, *et al*. Clinical management of asthma in 1999: the Asthma Insights and Reality in Europe (AIRE) study *European Respiratory Journal* 2000; **16(5)**: 802–7.

26 • Murray C J L, Lopez A D. Evidence based health policy: lessons from the global burden of disease study *Science* 1996; **274**: 740–3.

27 • Pearson MG, Bucknall CE (eds). *Measuring Clinical Outcome in Asthma: a patient-focused approach* London: Royal College of Physicians, 1999.

28 • Kinnersley P, Stott N, Peters T J, *et al*. The patient-centredness of consultations and outcome in primary care *British Journal of General Practice* 1999; **49**: 711–16.

29 • Kaplan S H, Greenfield S, Ware J E. Assessing the effects of physician–patient interactions on the outcomes of chronic disease *Medical Care* 1989; **27(Suppl. 3)**: S110–27.

30 • Towle A, Godolphin W. Framework for teaching and learning informed shared decision making *British Medical Journal* 1999; **319**: 766–71.

15

31 • Weston W W. Informed and shared decision-making: the crux of patient-centred care *Canadian Medical Association Journal* 2001; **165**: 438–9.

32 • Lorig K, Ritter P, Stewart A, *et al.* Chronic disease and self-management program. 2-year health status and health care utilization outcomes *Medical Care* 2001; **39(11)**: 1217–23.

33 • Education for Health. *Partners in Care: five steps to a better consultation* Warwick: Education for Health, 2007.

34 • Rimmer R, Quinn J. Audit of asthma care. Poster at Annual Conference of the National Centre for Clinical Audit, November 1998.

35 • Neville R G, Hoskins G, Smith B, *et al.* Observations on the structure, process and clinical outcomes of asthma care in general practice *British Journal of General Practice* 1996; **46**: 583–7.

36 • Smellie A, Campbell D, Bowie A. The impact of structured care on paediatric asthma management as assessed by audit. Poster at Annual Conference of the National Centre for Clinical Audit, November 1998.

37 • Holmes W F, Macfarlane J. Issues at the interface between primary and secondary care in the management of common respiratory disease *Thorax* 1999; **54(6)**: 538–9.

38 • Department of Health. *The NHS Plan*, London: DH, 2000.

39 • Pinnock H, Netuveli G, Price D, et al. General practitioners with a special interest in respiratory medicine: national survey of UK primary care organisations *BMC Health Services Research* 27 May 2005, doi: 10.1186 / 1472-6963-5-40.

Clinical examination

2

Yvonne Henderson, Simon Gregory and Stephen Holmes

Chapter aims

This book is aimed at those in GP training. It is therefore reasonable to assume that the reader is experienced in the clinical examination of the respiratory patient. Even the most experienced clinician can benefit from refreshing his or her knowledge and technique. This chapter is intended to help with this. If you are confident of your examination skills you might wish to skip this chapter.

Learning outcomes

▷ To refresh knowledge of how to examine the respiratory system.
▷ To revise the main findings of clinical significance from such examination.

Assessing the respiratory patient

Observation

Physical examination begins as the patient walks into the room.
　From the moment you meet that individual you should be noticing:

▷ whether he or she is distressed
▷ if he or she is breathless, able to complete a sentence in one breath
▷ his or her breathing pattern – rapid, shallow, deep, pursed lipped, sighing, etc.
▷ his or her colour and posture
▷ whether he or she appears to be in pain
▷ his or her facial expressions in reaction to things you have said
▷ his or her dress and grooming
▷ if there is any odour, e.g. cigarettes, alcohol, etc.

THE FACE

A bluish tinge to the tongue (except in black and Asian patients) indicates central cyanosis and hypoxaemia.

A sweet, fruity smell (likened to 'pear drops') to the breath might be a sign of diabetes. Halitosis is often a feature of bronchiectasis.

THE HANDS

FINGER CLUBBING

This is a non-specific clinical sign and the mechanism of its development is not understood. It occurs in a variety of chronic cardio-respiratory conditions, particularly bronchiectasis, lung cancer and diseases causing diffuse lung fibrosis. It is also a feature of congenital heart disease and can be found in cirrhosis and coeliac disease.

There is normally a slight 'angle' at the root of the nail bed. In clubbed fingers the nail bed is raised and this angle is lost. In advanced clubbing the finger tip will look bulbous and feel spongy (see Figure 2.1).

Figure 2.1 ○ *Finger clubbing*

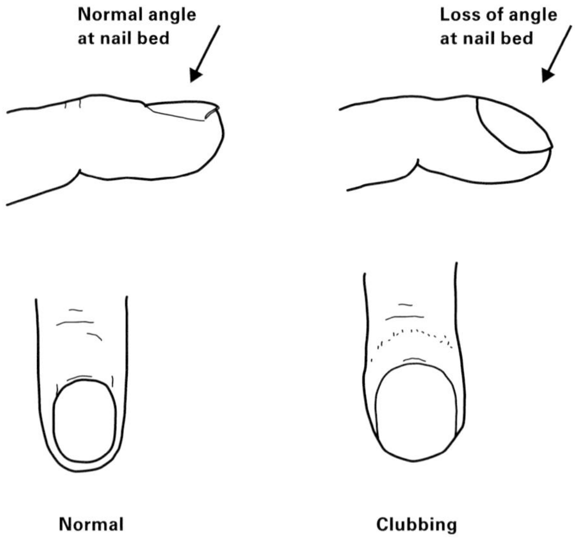

Normal angle at nail bed

Loss of angle at nail bed

Normal

Clubbing

Source: reproduced by kind permission of Education for Health.

WARMTH

Local peripheral vasoconstriction might give the hands a pallid or cyanosed appearance.

Carbon dioxide retention causes peripheral vascular dilation and enhances blood flow. In this case the hands might be strikingly warm.

COLOUR

Peripheral cyanosis can be innocent if the hands are cold, but if they are warm the peripheral circulation is likely to be good and the cyanosis will be a sign of hypoxaemia.

THE PULSE

It is vital to take the pulse whenever examining a respiratory patient. The trend to accept the pulse rate provided by the automated sphygmomanometer is not acceptable. The peripheral pulse should be palpated for rate, rhythm, volume and character. Without doing so subtleties will be missed, and arrhythmias are not indicated by automated machines. The irregularly irregular pulse of atrial fibrillation quickly explains, for example, a new onset of breathlessness. Whilst not scientific, the act of taking the pulse is also an important means of achieving touch, which creates contact and physically breaks down barriers with the patient.

There is a number of abnormal peripheral pulses.

▷ A small, weak pulse might indicate a low circulating volume, e.g. shock (when the pulse will also be rapid), but is also felt in heart failure or severe aortic stenosis.
▷ A strong, bounding pulse is sometimes felt in patients with anaemia, fever or hyperthyroidism. It is also sometimes present in carbon dioxide retention.
▷ A slow, bounding pulse might indicate heart block.
▷ A pulse that decreases in rate during inspiration and increases during expiration is termed a 'paradoxical' pulse. This is found in cardiac tamponade due to conditions such as restrictive pericarditis.

LOWER LIMBS AND ANKLES

Peripheral oedema will normally be detected in the lower limbs and ankles, but in an immobile patient this will be evident in the sacrum.

Unilateral oedema might be due to varicose veins in the affected leg, but could also be a sign of deep vein thrombosis.

THE SKIN

ERYTHEMA NODOSUM

This is characterised by raised, tender red swellings over the shins. They occur in crops, often over several weeks. Joint pains and fever might also be present. The condition is associated with sarcoidosis, but can also occur with pulmonary tuberculosis and streptococcal infection.

SKIN NODULES

These are sometimes seen in sarcoidosis, and are associated with metastatic carcinoma.

THE CHEST

SHAPE

A kyphosis is a rounded thoracic convexity and is often seen in elderly patients, particularly women.

A scoliosis (a lateral curvature of the spine) can occur as a compensation for another structural abnormality, such as a shortened leg – a functional scoliosis. This is usually benign. Scoliosis is often, however, associated with a rotation of the vertebra – a kyphoscoliosis. When this is severe or progressive it can seriously interfere with respiratory movements.

A 'barrel chest' is a typical finding in obstructive airways disease. The thorax is over-inflated and the anteroposterior diameter of the chest is increased.

CHEST SYMMETRY

The hemithoraces will be unequal if there is a kyphoscoliosis, but pathology in the underlying organs can also destroy the symmetry of the chest. Fibrosis affecting one lung will reduce the volume of the hemithorax on that side.

Respiratory rate

It is vital to carefully count the respiratory rate. It is best to do this in a manner that does not alert the patient as to what you are doing, because this will alter his or her rate. Changes in the respiratory rate can be amongst the earliest signs of a serious deterioration in health and its value is often underestimated. This can be especially so in children, in whom the respiratory rate can be a vital sign of serious disease, and for emergency action, such as the need for hospital admission.

NB: special skills are required to examine children, especially ill ones. An adaptable and opportunistic approach is vital. For example, you may wish to listen to a child's chest before examining its ears as a screaming child makes chest examination rather tricky.

Action point

Look at the NICE guidelines on *Feverish Illness in Children* and the RCGP/BMA/DH flu pandemic guidance to understand the importance of respiratory rate in assessing a sick child.

RESPIRATORY MOVEMENT

Impaired movement on one side suggests a problem in the underlying lung or pleura.

ACCESSORY MUSCLES

The use of accessory muscles at rest is always abnormal. Retraction of the lower costal interspaces during inspiration is a sign of severe obstructive airways disease.

Palpation

The trachea

The trachea should be central. It can be pushed to one side by masses in the neck, but deviation is also an important indicator of:

▷ a mass in the mediastinum
▷ collapse of a lung due to pneumothorax
▷ extensive consolidation.

Respiratory expansion

The movement should be symmetrical. Unequal expansion could be due to a variety of pathologies in the underlying lung and pleura, including:

▷ fibrosis
▷ consolidation
▷ pleural effusion

▷ pleuritic pain leading to splinting
▷ one-sided bronchial obstruction.

Poor expansion in the presence of a hyperinflated thorax is commonly seen in chronic obstructive pulmonary disease (COPD).

Figure 2.2 ○ **Position of the hands when feeling for respiratory expansion**

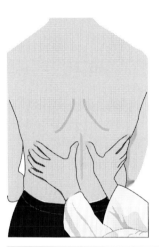

Source: reproduced by kind permission of Education for Health.

Fremitus

Fremitus is the term used to describe vibrations from the voice transmitted through the bronchopulmonary tree to the chest wall. It is reduced in:

▷ COPD
▷ obstruction of the bronchus
▷ pleural effusion or pneumothorax, or infiltrating tumour such as mesothelioma.

It is increased when the underlying lobe is consolidated.

Cardiac apex

The characteristics of the apical impulse help determine the size of the left ventricle.

The cardiac apex is normally felt in the left midclavicular line in the fourth or fifth interspace. It might be difficult to locate in a very obese patient or when the thorax is hyperinflated (barrel chest).

Figure 2.3 ○ *Where to feel for fremitus on the posterior and anterior chest wall*

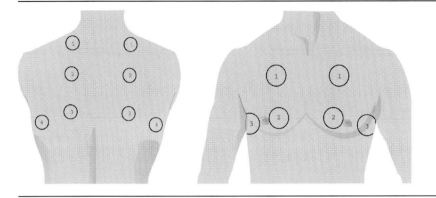

Source: reproduced by kind permission of Education for Health.

A particularly strong apical impulse, or an impulse that is felt far to the left of the midclavicular line, might indicate an enlarged left ventricle. A loud heart murmur might produce a palpable 'thrill'.

Jugular venous pressure

Jugular venous pressure (JVP) is a reflection of pressure in the right atrium and the central venous pressure.

JVP is elevated in right-sided heart failure and cor pulmonale.

Percussion

The percussion note is dull over solid organs, such as the liver or heart, and resonant over aerated lung. In conditions such as COPD where the lung is over-inflated the percussion note will be hyper-resonant and the dull percussion note usually found over the heart might be lost. The percussion note will also change if the lung is consolidated or there is a pleural effusion or pneumothorax.

The diaphragm is pushed downwards when the lungs are hyperinflated. If the percussion note changes at a higher level than you would expect, this could indicate a pleural effusion.

Figure 2.4 ○ *Areas for percussion and auscultation of the chest*

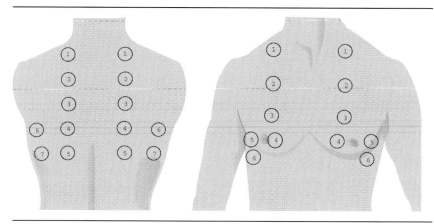

Source: reproduced by kind permission of Education for Health.

Auscultation

Listening to the lungs

Listening with a stethoscope augments the information gained from observation and percussion of the chest wall.

Listen to the sounds generated by breathing (the breath sounds) and any additional sounds, and if appropriate listen to the sound of the patient's voice as it is transmitted through the lungs and chest wall (transmitted voice sounds).

BREATH SOUNDS

There are three basic, normal breath sounds. They differ in intensity and pitch, and the duration of their inspiratory and expiratory phases. They are as follows:

1 ▷ **vesicular breath sounds** • these are heard over most of the lungs. They are soft, low-pitched sounds. They are heard throughout inspiration and continue into expiration without a silent phase. They fade about a third of the way through expiration.

2 ▷ **bronchovesicular sounds** • these are heard mainly over the first and second interspaces anteriorly and between the scapulae posteriorly. The inspiratory and expiratory phases are about equal in length and occasionally separated by a short interval of silence.

3 ▷ **bronchial sounds** • these are sometimes not heard at all and are only audible over the manubrium. They are louder and higher pitched than the other breath sounds. Expiratory sounds continue for longer than the inspiratory sounds.

Breath sounds generated in the trachea are very loud and are only heard over the trachea.

Breath sounds are generally reduced in severe emphysema and there might be local areas of reduced sounds over bullae. Breath sounds will be absent or reduced in pneumothorax or pleural effusion. When a lung lobe is poorly ventilated, e.g. when the bronchus supplying that area is blocked by tumour, the breath sounds will be reduced.

When the lungs are consolidated, or where there are large cavities, the harsh, high-pitched bronchial sounds will be transmitted and will be heard with a stethoscope placed over the affected area.

ADDITIONAL SOUNDS

There are four basic types of additional sound:

1 ▷ **crackles** (sometimes also called râles) • these are intermittent and non-musical. Each sound is of brief duration. They can be described as fine (soft, high-pitched and brief – less than 10 milliseconds) or coarse (louder, lower-pitched, lasting for longer – 20–30 milliseconds). Fine crackles are sometimes likened to the noise of Velcro being slowly torn apart. Fine, late inspiratory crackles are a feature of pulmonary fibrosis. Crackles can also be heard in congestive heart failure

2 ▷ **wheezes** • these sounds are relatively high-pitched and continuous. They occur when the airway is narrowed. Each sound is notably longer than a crackle. Where airway obstruction is widespread each obstructed airway produces a sound that is slightly differently pitched. This gives an overall musical and 'polyphonic' quality to the wheeze. Obstruction in a single, larger airway will give a 'monophonic' quality to the wheeze. In asthma and COPD widespread polyphonic wheezes may be heard on expiration

3 ▷ **rhonchi** • like wheezes, rhonchi are continuous but they are lower in pitch and have a 'snoring' quality. They are associated with secretions in the airways and will often clear on coughing

4 ▷ **pleural rub** • this sound is generated by two layers of abnormal pleura (e.g. inflamed or traumatised) moving over each other. It is a 'creaking' sound that you might confuse with crackles. It is usually heard in a confined area of the chest; crackles are often more widespread.

Listening to the heart

There are four main auscultatory areas:

▷ second right interspace close to the sternum (aortic valve)
▷ second left interspace close to the sternum (pulmonary valve)
▷ fifth right interspace close to the sternum (tricuspid valve)
▷ at the apex (mitral valve) (see Figure 2.5).

Figure 2.5 ○ *Auscultatory areas of the heart*

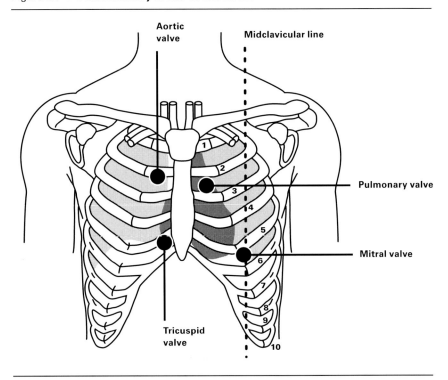

Source: reproduced by kind permission of Education for Health.

S1 and S2 (the 'lub–dup' heart sounds) are generated by the heart valves closing during the cardiac cycle. S1 to S2 occur close together in the systolic phase and are followed by a brief pause (diastolic) before the S1, S2 sequence begins again.

Murmurs are described as:

▷ **systolic** • occurring between S1 (lub) and S2 (dup)
▷ **diastolic** • occurring between S2 (dup) and S1 (lub).

Systolic murmurs

These can last throughout the entire S1 to S2 period (pansystolic) or can occur between S1 and S2 with a brief gap between the murmur and the heart sound (midsystolic). Occasionally a third variation can be heard: the late systolic murmur. There is a gap after S1 and the murmur persists into S2.

Diastolic murmurs

These are almost always pathological. They are associated with incompetence of the aortic valve or stenosis of the mitral valve.

Additional heart sounds

These are the result of:

▷ vibrations caused by rapid filling of the ventricles (the third heart sound – S3), often heard in acute pulmonary embolism
▷ atria contracting to fill the ventricles against abnormal resistance (the fourth heart sound – S4), suggestive of coronary heart disease.

Smoking
Its impact

3

Roswyn Hakesley-Brown

A cigarette is 'a euphemism for a cleverly crafted product that delivers just the right amount of nicotine to keep its user addicted for life, before killing [that] person'.[1]

Chapter aims

▷ To enhance the understanding of the impact of smoking on the health economy and its relevance for general practice.
▷ To facilitate the integration of nicotine addiction management into the general practice enterprise, including the utilisation of smoking cessation interventions where appropriate.

Learning outcomes

▷ To identify and manage primary contact with patients who are addicted to tobacco.
▷ To identify and manage primary contact with patients who are passive smokers.
▷ To demonstrate a consistent, evidence-based approach to smoking cessation interventions.
▷ To co-ordinate the delivery of smoking cessation interventions with other primary care health professionals including practice nurses, district nurses, public health nurses, health visitors, school nurses, advanced nurse practitioners, healthcare assistants, physiotherapists, pharmacists, alternative therapists and behavioural psychologists.

Initial self-assessment

Which of the following statements about smoking are true?

1 ▷ Smoking has decreased amongst males and females over the last five decades.

2 ▷ Most smokers want to stop smoking.

3 ▷ More than 200,000 people die from smoking-related diseases in the UK each year.

4 ▷ Smokers can save upwards of £2000 p.a. by giving up smoking.

5 ▷ The prevalence of smoking has not reduced in countries that have banncd smoking in public places.

Key ▶ **T T F** (more than 100,000), **T F** (there is good evidence that it has reduced).

Introduction

Respiratory problems are the most common cause for patients seeing their general practitioner (GP) and for emergency medical admission to hospital. Furthermore, smoking cessation advice is a key element of health promotion activity in primary care.[2]

Eight million people suffer from respiratory disease in the UK, with one third of the population visiting their general practice at least once a year with a respiratory condition.[3]

The link between tobacco use and respiratory ill health is well established.[4] When this is also linked to the level of general practice consultations/hospital admissions for respiratory problems, it becomes clear that the GP and the primary care team are in pole positions to play a major role in reducing the negative impact that smoking has on public health. However, this negative impact is further expanded by the fact that smoking is also responsible for other pathologies, in addition to those affecting the respiratory system. As the Director General of the World Health Organization, Dr Gro Harlem Brundtland, points out:

More people smoke today than at any other time in human history. One person dies every ten seconds due to smoking-related diseases.[5]

Understanding the impact of smoking on the respiratory health of the primary care patient community is an essential precursor to developing an appropriate primary care infrastructure for the effective delivery of smoking cessation interventions. The health benefits are incontestable and have immediate as well as long-term effects. Paradoxically,

tobacco is the only legally available consumer product which kills people when it is entirely used as intended.[6]

That is, correct usage of the product has the ultimate potential outcome of causing the death of the user.

The position of doctors, particularly frontline workers such as GPs and their teams, is highly influential in the fight against the tobacco epidemic. That great and well-known protagonist in this area, the late Sir Richard Doll, recognised this when he wrote:

the greater contribution that all doctors can make is … through direct contact with their patients to improve long term health and through their professional organisations to achieve the same objectives by affecting government policy.[7]

GPs thus have the unique opportunity to work at both strategic and operational levels. This is a powerful mix for making a difference to the health of the nation.

Epidemiology and politics of smoking

Tobacco will be the largest preventable cause of ill health that most doctors will meet.[8] It is claimed that there are just three risk factors (tobacco use, lack of physical activity and an unhealthy diet) that are responsible for the four chronic diseases (40 per cent of all cancers, heart disease, stroke and type II diabetes), which, in turn, are responsible for over 50 per cent of deaths worldwide.[9]

Placing the tobacco epidemic into a global political socioeconomic context is an important aspect of understanding about smoking. There is a wealth of evidence available that illustrates the increasing penetration by tobacco multinational companies, e.g. British American Tobacco (BAT), into the economic marketplaces of developing countries such as Malawi and China.[10] Tobacco use is declining in the developed world, assisted by the rise of government tobacco control legislation such as:

▷ smoke-free public areas and workplaces
▷ control of underage sale of tobacco products
▷ controls over the promotion and advertising of tobacco products
▷ preventing illegal imports of tobacco (usually hand rolled)
▷ taxation of tobacco
▷ consumer information on packaging.

Tobacco companies have to find new marketplaces. In addition, they are vehemently opposed to any form of tobacco control, and will attempt to subvert any form of state interference in the marketing of their products. This is evidenced in the release of previously confidential internal documents forcibly released for litigation in the USA. Tobacco companies prefer to rely on the mantra of 'self-regulation' rather than state legislation. However, the observation that successful tobacco control means that sales of tobacco will fall is comfortingly apt.[8]

Understanding the epidemiological map, as well as the political influences relevant to the issues of tobacco use, is also essential in dealing with the impact of smoking on the public health community.

The supporting scientific evidence for tobacco as a major source of disease is huge. In the twentieth century 100 million people died from tobacco-related diseases. It is estimated that 1 billion deaths will be attributed to smoking in the twenty-first century.[5] Albeit that 70 per cent of these deaths are likely to take place in developing countries, this leaves no room for complacency in the UK for a number of both moral and economic reasons, not least of which is the issue of global migration and mobility. Although the evidence suggests that ethnic minority groups in the UK appear to smoke less than the UK population as a whole,[8] the figures for newly arrived immigrants might look rather different. A further important consideration is the fact that the large tobacco conglomerates are now targeting the developing world for both tobacco marketing purposes and cigarette manufacture.[11] Responding to the healthcare needs of minority ethnic populations is a major responsibility for GPs, who need to demonstrate a high level of culturally sensitive competence and awareness.

Despite the decline of tobacco use in the developed world, smoking continues to be the largest preventable cause of premature death.[8] In the United Kingdom (UK), male smoking (aged over 15) has gradually declined from 61 per cent in 1960 to 26 per cent in 2004. Smoking amongst females has similarly declined from 42 per cent in 1960 to 23 per cent in 2004. In addition, 56 per cent of people setting a date for smoking cessation had still quit after four weeks during 2004/5.[12] Most smokers want to stop smoking.

Male smokers generally smoke more cigarettes per day than females (14.5 as opposed to 13.3). They also have a tendency to smoke higher-tar cigarettes.[13, 14]

From a socioeconomic perspective, those in managerial/professional occupations smoke less than those in manual jobs. Levels of educational achievement are also significant in smoking prevalence. Low educational achievement in children has been found to be associated with increased smoking.[15] The World Health Organization (WHO) predicts that 200–300 million of today's children and adolescents will eventually die as a result of smoking.[16]

The fact that 8 per cent of male and 6 per cent of female physicians in the UK smoke gives some pause for thought in relation to the quality of social responsibility that health professionals display in relation to the provision of positive health promotion role models.[5] Seen as sources of reliable information and advice, doctors are also exemplars to the rest of the community.[8] In addition, physicians and nurses who were smokers were more proactive in delivering smoking cessation counselling and advice to patients, when they themselves had taken part in a smoking cessation study.[17] Having healthcare teams with good representation from ex-smokers bodes well for the introduction of successful smoking cessation intervention strategies.

There are also regional variations in smoking prevalence, usually relating to socioeconomic factors, with the south and western UK regions having a lower smoking prevalence than the northwest of England.[18]

Action learning point

Review a general practice population of your choice (e.g. a training placement) in relation to the following:

▶ geographical location
▶ age profile
▶ gender distribution
▶ socioeconomic status
▶ ethnic minority representation.

Estimate the likely prevalence of tobacco use.

Stigma – smoking and smoking-related diseases

Smokers can often be recognised by nicotine staining of the digits, a husky voice, a persistent, productive cough (sometimes accompanied by breathlessness and wheezing), facial wrinkling unrelated to age and a general aura of smoke carried on clothes and breath.

The kind of tobacco products that are consumed can variously include not only the most commonly used cigarette but also:

▷ **chewing tobacco** • sometimes called 'spit' tobacco because it requires saliva to activate the ingredients such as betel leaves, lime, etc.
▷ **nasal snuff** • a fine tobacco powder that is 'snorted' (not to be confused with cocaine!)
▷ **bidis** • hand-made cigarettes with strong flavouring, such as cloves, added
▷ **hookahs** • a water pipe that draws smoke through flavoured water, common in the Middle and Far East. However, according to a national broadsheet, this form of tobacco consumption is increasing in popularity for young Europeans[19]

▷ **Skol Bandits** • tobacco sachets for chewing, produced in the USA
▷ **cigars/cigarillos** • a more expensive variant of the cigarette usually produced from Cuban tobacco, often associated with famous figures such as Winston Churchill.

The rise of smoke-free public places might have a downside in that smokers might turn to smoke-free tobacco use. We might, therefore, see an increase in the use of chewing tobacco and nasal snuff as a result of these environmental changes in tobacco prohibition.

The evidence that tobacco use continues to be dangerous to health has already been demonstrated as compelling.[20–22] The smoke from burning tobacco contains over 4000 lethal gaseous components such as:

▷ acetaldehyde (found in paint stripper)
▷ formaldehyde (preservative for tissue specimens)
▷ carbon monoxide (car exhaust fumes)
▷ benzene (used in some insecticides).

There are also lethal solids in tobacco smoke in the form of particles such as:

▷ tar, containing carcinogens, polycyclic aromatic hydrocarbons (PAHs), dioxins and nitrosamines
▷ nicotine, which mimics the naturally occurring chemical messenger, acetylcholine (ACh).

Whilst the first five examples are highly toxic and have a toxic effect on most body systems including the respiratory system, it is the latter, nicotine, that is responsible for the tobacco addiction. This is what makes the habit so hard to 'kick'.[23,24] It really is a case of 'addiction leading to affliction'. If you look after the 'pennies' of addiction, it is more likely that the 'pounds' of affliction will look after themselves! Thereby lies the cost … and the saving, not only in terms of health economics, but also in terms of the social costs of human misery.

Action learning point

Refer to the section on clinical management in the RCGP Curriculum for Specialty Training for General Practice (www.rcgp-curriculum.org.uk/rcgp_-_gp_curriculum_documents/gp_curriculum_statements.aspx). Focus on curriculum statements 15.3 (*Drug and Alcohol Problems*) and 15.7 (*Neurological Problems*), and identify four physiological contributors to nicotine addiction:

▶ nicotinic acetylcholine receptors
▶ ventral tegmental segment (VTA)

▶ nucleus accumbens (NAcc)
▶ dopamine.

This more detailed physiological understanding of nicotine addiction is essential for the support of patients who are trying to give up. *Giving up is very hard to do!*

Approximately 106,000 people die from smoking-related diseases each year in the UK. That works out at about 12 people every hour.[25] The following proportions of deaths are attributed to smoking:[26]

▷ cardiovascular disease, 31 per cent
▷ lung cancer, 25 per cent
▷ chronic obstructive pulmonary disease (COPD), 20 per cent
▷ other cancers, 13 per cent
▷ pneumonia, 9 per cent
▷ digestive disorders, 2 per cent.

That is over 50 per cent of deaths caused by the effect of smoking on the respiratory system. Smokers are 15 times more likely to contract lung cancer than non-smokers.[27]

COPD, including both emphysema and chronic bronchitis, accounts for over one fifth of all smoking-related deaths.[21] COPD results from smoke damage to both the central and peripheral airways, extending as far as the alveoli and capillaries.

The carcinogens in tobacco smoke are dispersed throughout the body and can be linked to other types of cancer, as well as those affecting the respiratory tract.[28] Therefore, there is a high 'value added' dimension to investing in general practice-based smoking cessation interventions.

Health gain cycle applied to smoking cessation

Smoking cessation is the single most important action people can take to improve both their current and future health.[7] Ideally, cessation is most beneficial before the age of 35 before any smoking-related diseases manifest themselves. However, smokers who smoke longer and stop later will still improve their life expectancy.

The Action on Smoking and Health (ASH) fact sheet graphically describes the health benefits when people stop smoking (see Table 3.1).

Table 3.1 ○ *Health benefits of smoking cessation*

Time since quitting	Beneficial health changes
20 minutes	Blood pressure and pulse returns to normal
8 hours	Nicotine and carbon monoxide levels in blood reduce by 50%, oxygen levels return to normal
24 hours	Carbon monoxide is eliminated from the body. Mucus and other smoking debris reduces in the lungs
48 hours	Body is nicotine free. Considerable improvement of taste and smell
72 hours	Respiration is less laboured. Airways relax and energy levels increase
2–12 weeks	Circulation improves
3–9 months	Coughs, wheezing and breathing problems improve as lung function increases by up to 10%
1 year	Risk of myocardial infarction falls to approximately half that of a smoker
10 years	Risk of lung cancer falls to half that of a smoker
15 years	Risk of myocardial infarction falls to the same as someone who has never smoked

Source: modified from Action on Smoking and Health.[29]

The downside of smoking cessation for smokers is that they will experience a number of nicotine withdrawal symptoms, which will need careful management and sensitive support from the healthcare team. These symptoms will include both physical and mental changes such as:

▷ irritability/aggression (usually for less than 4 weeks)
▷ depression (less than 4 weeks)
▷ restlessness (less than 4 weeks)
▷ poor concentration (less than 2 weeks)
▷ increased appetite (more than 10 weeks)
▷ light-headedness (less than 48 hours)
▷ insomnia (less than 1 week)
▷ cravings (more than 2 weeks).[29]

Understanding these smoking cessation side effects will facilitate a proactive approach to interventions to ensure increased success rates in cessation uptake.

Smoking cessation

The evidence suggests that smokers are more motivated to accept advice about smoking when it is related to an existing condition, which may not necessarily be associated with smoking.[30] Establishing the smoking status of patients, including child patients who a) may already be acquiring the habit or b) be living in households where passive smoking is a health hazard, is an important dimension of the individual patient record and the practice profile. Patients might be described as either a smoker, non-smoker, recent ex-smoker or living/working in a smoke-contaminated environment. This evidence will constitute a significant part of the evidence on which to base the development of intervention strategies for both individuals and groups of patients. Establishing smoking status should be seen as being as routine as establishing vital signs and as important.

The management of the initial assessment is crucial to the success of any intervention. The decision to stop smoking can only come from the patients themselves. An acceptable opening question from the GP to ascertain where the patient is in the cycle of stopping is 'Have you ever thought of giving up tobacco?' There is a number of responses that patients can make to this question:

▷ does not want to stop smoking
▷ not interested in stopping at this time, but might be in future
▷ would like to stop smoking now.

Patients for whom smoking cessation has never been a consideration might take a little longer to embark on the cessation journey. Indeed they might never take that first step, and that is their choice. However, leaving the topic open for future discussion, with offers of support, could prove to be a very attractive option to the patient. A note should be made in his or her documentation to reassess the situation within the next 12 months.

However, most people would like to stop. The cycle of stopping has several stages:

▷ **stage 1** • thinking about stopping
▷ **stage 2** • preparing to stop; planning contributes to success
▷ **stage 3** • actually stopping by setting a definite quit date
▷ **stage 4** • continuing the cessation by changing approach to smoking and making appropriate lifestyle changes.

Stage 5 • is 'relapsing': people might fail to stop several times, for a number of reasons. These reasons need to be reflected on and lessons learnt ready for the next attempt.[31]

NB: further understanding of and guidance to managing this cycle can be obtained from the RCGP publication *The Patient–Doctor Consultation in Primary Care*.[32]

There is a number of examples of how this first encounter with a smoker can be managed, such as:[24]

▷ discussing the risks of smoking, particularly in relation to the current personal health scenario

▷ discussing the general risks to health and the effect on longevity

▷ discussing smoking in relation to other family members, e.g. a young child with asthma or a premature baby

▷ highlighting the amount of money that can be saved, e.g. a 20-a-day smoker can save upwards of £2000 a year (and with each budget – climbing!). Collecting the savings in a jar and watching it grow can be hugely motivational, particularly if plans are in place to spend it on something desirable such as a holiday abroad.

Opportunistic brief interventions can be a very good starting point for all members of the general practice team, including the following:

▷ **general practitioner** • most consultations with smokers are opportunities for advice and possible intervention/referral, e.g. smoking clinic

▷ **practice nurse** • all routine consultations including screening for blood pressure etc.

▷ **dentist** • all routine dental checks with referral to the general practice team if appropriate

▷ **pharmacist** • relate to and refer on, if appropriate, any client presenting prescriptions for respiratory conditions or demonstrating an interest in nicotine replacement therapy

▷ **physiotherapist** • patients presenting for physiotherapy treatment, particularly respiratory problems, can be offered advice and referral

▷ **receptionist** • might observe patient reading smoking cessation literature/notices in the waiting room. Could offer further information in support of interest, e.g. information about free NHS treatment for smokers, smoking cessation clinics, etc.

Once an evaluation of interest in quitting has been carried out, a more detailed assessment needs to be undertaken about the patient's smoking history. In addition to the Read code for never smoked, ex-smoker, smoker, the practice might have also developed a specific electronic assessment form for documenting this. This could include information such as:

▷ age at which smoking commenced
▷ reason for starting to smoke (e.g. trigger)
▷ what kind of tobacco product, e.g. cigarettes, tipped or roll-ups, etc.
▷ how many smoked per day when patient began smoking
▷ has smoking been continuous since then and, if not, what changes have been made to smoking habit and why.

The next important step to be taken by a member of the practice team (this does not necessarily have to be the GP) is the assessment of tobacco dependence, in order to give the most appropriate smoking cessation advice. A recognised measure is the Fagerströmt Test for Nicotine Dependence (FTND) (see Table 3.2).[33]

Table 3.2 ○ *Fagerström Test for Nicotine Dependence*

Question	Answer	Score
How soon after waking do you smoke your first cigarette?	Within 5 minutes	3
	6–30 minutes	2
	31–60 minutes	1
	>60 minutes	0
Do you find it difficult to refrain from smoking in places where it is forbidden?	Yes	1
	No	0
Which cigarette would you hate to give up most?	The first one in the morning	1
	Others	0
How many cigarettes per day do you smoke?	≤10	0
	11–20	1
	21–30	2
	≥31	3
Do you smoke more frequently during the first hours of waking than during the rest of the day?	Yes	1
	No	0
Do you smoke if you are so ill that you are in bed for most of the day?	Yes	1
	No	0

Source: Heatherton T F, Koslowski LT, Frecker R C. The Fagerström tolerance questionnaire *British Journal of Addiction* 1991; **86(9)**: 1119–27. Copyright© 1991 Blackwell Publishing Ltd. Reproduced with permission of Blackwell Publishing Ltd.

Note: scores are totalled to give a single value. A threshold of 7 is used to divide smokers into high- and low-dependence categories.

A score of 7 and over indicates a high level of addiction that is likely to need more robust interventions. The WHO European recommendations (2001) for the treatment of tobacco dependence define brief interventions as the five 'As':[34]

▷ **Ask** • about smoking at every opportunity
▷ **Advise** • all smokers to stop in a personalised and appropriate manner
▷ **Assess** • motivation to change
▷ **Assist** • the smoker to stop
▷ **Arrange** • follow-up if possible.

Assisting the smoker to stop begins with taking a quick smoking history, and then planning, implementing and evaluating the cessation process. This includes:

▷ reviewing past attempts to stop – what helped and the barriers to success
▷ planning ahead in the light of this experience; discussing strategies to overcome problems such as withdrawal symptoms or social pressure to smoke
▷ advising smoker to inform family, friends and colleagues to obtain support, particularly exhorting those who smoke not to subvert attempts at cessation!
▷ identifying and setting a quit date and obtaining agreement to stick to it. Advise the smoker not to buy too many cigarettes the day before the quit date!
▷ planning how the smoker will manage social occasions etc. where the risk of being offered cigarettes is high
▷ encouraging the use of nicotine replacement therapy (NRT), bupropion and varenicline
▷ arranging follow-up for approximately a week's time for monitoring, evaluation and further advice (modified from Percival et al.).[23]

Incorporating some psycho-social understanding at this point is also useful by utilising, for instance, the concept of locus of control in identifying the smokers' health beliefs in terms of either:[35]

▷ belief that they have control over the state of their own health (internal locus of control)

or

▷ belief that prevention of illness is outside their control (external locus of control).

Understanding where the health locus of control lies with individual smokers might be helpful in deciding which kind of interventions would be most useful.

Good preparation for quitting adds to the likelihood of smoking cessation success. This can be enhanced by encouraging patients to use the NHS

Helpline (0800 022 4 332) or visit the website at www.gosmokefree.co.uk for extra support. The free NHS booklet[36] also contains useful advice for effective preparation, which encourages the smoker to write down what he or she can do to address the following issues:

▷ avoiding temptation
▷ getting support
▷ changing the way that smoking is perceived
▷ coping with cravings
▷ creating specific activities for the first week of smoking cessation.

It generally takes 5–6 attempts before a smoker finally succeeds in quitting. Care should be exercised in how using this kind of information is managed. It could be perceived as permission to fail if given before the quit date (fulfilling expectations). Alternatively, at the first quit failure, some indication could be given that to fail is not unusual in the initial stages of attempting to quit.

GPs can both create and utilise a number of services and motivational devices to support the brief smoking interventions provided by the practice team. These include:

▷ regular carbon monoxide monitoring for checking progress *and* covert relapses
▷ the creation of a Smoking Cessation Clinic or local 'stop smoking group' led by practice nurses
▷ telephone counselling
▷ effective use of pharmaceutical support for NRT (gum, patches, microtabs, lozenges, nasal sprays and inhalers), bupropion, hydrochloride, etc.
▷ refer to the local NHS Smoking Service (which provides specialist treatment for smokers wishing to stop) or the NHS Smoking Helpline. There is also an Asian Tobacco Helpline, available in Urdu, Punjabi, etc.
▷ refer for complementary therapy if appropriate (hypnosis, acupuncture, etc.)
▷ encourage patients to keep a smoking diary
▷ maintain availability of free literature such as *Giving Up for Life*.[31]

Patients who fail their attempts at quitting, or do not wish to quit at all, might be offered advice on cutting down their tobacco consumption. Every year, 33 per cent of smokers try to cut down.[37] However, these smokers tend to engage in *compensatory smoking* (smoking more intensively by drawing harder/longer on the cigarette, puffing it more frequently and smoking down to the filter).[38] Changing to a lower-tar cigarette also produces the same compensatory effect. Cutting down might need to be supported by

NRT with a view to stopping completely at a future date. Cutting down alone is unlikely to bring any real health benefits.[39]

The reported perceived benefits of smoking to the user must not be under-estimated.[24] These include:

▷ coping with stress
▷ relief of boredom
▷ enjoyment
▷ facilitating concentration
▷ socialising and avoiding discomfort
▷ weight control.

Offering alternative strategies for replacing cigarettes as a contributor to the above can be a useful part of the smoking cessation advice portfolio.

If a patient relapses and returns to smoking, allow a suitable period of time to elapse before beginning the next attempt at cessation. This will give the smoker time to reflect on what it was that triggered him or her into restarting the habit and take the necessary steps to avoid such triggers in future. People give a wide variety of reasons for returning to smoking such as:

▷ I thought I could just have one cigarette
▷ I had a stressful day
▷ I needed a cigarette to deal with the pressure I've been under
▷ I didn't have a planned programme of cessation to keep me on track.

Successful smoking cessation is built on positive partnerships between the smokers and the health professionals. The smoker's autonomy must be respected with the professional partner taking a supporting and advisory role. Implied criticism of the smoker might be very counter-productive.

Passive and occupational smoking

There is robust evidence to support the thesis that exposure to environmental tobacco smoke (ETS) or passive smoking/second-hand smoke can also seriously affect the respiratory systems of non-smokers.[40-42] Second-hand smoke is divided into two types a) 'mainstream' smoke, exhaled by the smoker, and b) 'side-stream' smoke, which is emitted by a burning cigarette. Exposure to second-hand smoke can cause:

▷ irritation of the eyes, nose and throat
▷ headaches, dizziness and nausea
▷ exacerbation of asthma and allergies

▷ an increase, in the case of long-term exposure, in the risk of lung cancer by 10–30 per cent. The entertainer Roy Castle died of lung cancer; the cancer was commonly thought to be caused by passive inhalation of smoke whilst working in pubs and clubs at the outset of his career
▷ children to become prone to a number of conditions including chest infections, asthma, coughs, colds and wheezes
▷ children to be off sick from school more often. Their education can be compromised.

Conclusion

Perhaps the guru of smoking-related disease evidence, the late Richard Doll – the British physiologist and epidemiologist who was the first to prove that smoking causes lung cancer and increases the rate of ischaemic heart disease – should be allowed the final word:

Patients turn to doctors for absolution not exhortation, and few have been trained in the art of prevention as effectively as in the art of cure. Both require art as well as scientific knowledge to achieve their aim.[7]

By understanding about the impact of smoking on health and putting in place strategies to reduce those risks, the GP has a real opportunity to make a real difference to the real health of the nation.

Resources

The Oxford Health Alliance • **www.oxha.org**.

References

1 • Brundtland GH. Speech at the International Council of Nurses Centennial Conference, London, 1999.

2 • Royal College of General Practitioners. *Respiratory Problems* (curriculum statement 15.8) London: RCGP, 2008.

3 • British Thoracic Society. *Burden of Lung Disease: a statistics report from the British Thoracic Society* London: BTS, 2001. www.brit-thoracic.org.uk/Portals/0/Library/BTS%20 Publications/burden_of_lung_disease.pdf [accessed January 2009].

4 • Boyle P. Cancer, cigarette smoking and premature death in Europe: a review including the recommendations of European Cancer Experts Consensus Meeting. Helsinki, Finland, October 1996 *Lung Cancer* 1997; **17**: 1–60.

5 • Brundtland G H. Foreword. In: Mackay J, Erikson M. *The Tobacco Atlas* Geneva: World Health Organization, 2002.

6 • Walton J, Barondess J A, Lock S (eds). *The Oxford Medical Companion* Oxford: Oxford University Press, 1994.

7 • Doll R. Foreword. In: D Simpson. *Doctors and Tobacco: medicine's big challenge* London: The Tobacco Control Resource Centre at the British Medical Association, 2000.

8 • Simpson D. *Doctors and Tobacco: medicine's big challenge* London: Tobacco Control Resource Centre at the British Medical Association, 2000.

9 • Oxford Health Alliance. *Confronting the Epidemic of Chronic Disease* London. Oxford Health Alliance, 2006, www.oxha.org/knowledge/publications/oha_basic-brochure-d14fb.pdf [accessed January 2009] .

10 • American Cancer Society, International Union Against Cancer and the World Health Organization. *Tobacco Control Country Profile* Geneva: WHO, 2003.

11 • Macdonald T H. *Third World Health: hostage to First World wealth* Oxford: Radcliffe Publishing, 2005.

12 • Department of Health. *Health Profile of England* London: DH, 2004.

13 • NatCen. *Health Survey for England 2003: latest trends* London: National Centre for Social Research, 2004.

14 • Office for National Statistics. *Living in Britain: results from the 1996 General Household Survey* London: The Stationery Office, 1997.

15 • Barton J. *Young Teenagers and Smoking in 1997* London: Health Education Authority, 1998.

16 • Whyte F, Kearney N. *Enhancing the Nurse's Role in Tobacco Control* London: The Tobacco Control Resource Centre at the British Medical Association, 2000.

17 • Puska P M J, Barrueco M, Roussos C, *et al.* The participation of health professionals in a smoking-cessation programme positively influences the smoking cessation advice given to patients *Journal of Clinical Practice* 2005; **59(4)**: 447–52.

18 • Department of Health. *Smoking Kills: a white paper on tobacco* London: The Stationery Office, 1998.

19 • Expert traveller: how to ... smoke a hookah pipe *Observer* 10 December 2006 (Escape Supplement): 3.

20 • US Department of Health and Human Services. *The Health Benefits of Smoking Cessation: a report of the Surgeon General* Atlanta, GA: USDHHS, Centres for Disease Control and Prevention, National Centre for Chronic Disease Prevention and Health Promotion, Office on Smoking and Health, 2004.

21 • Peto R, Lopez A, Boreham J, *et al. Mortality in Smoking in Developed Countries 1950–2000* (second edn) Oxford: Oxford University Press, 2004.

22 • Doll R. Uncovering the effects of smoking: historical perspective *Statistical Methods in Medical Research* 1998; **7**: 87–117.

23 • Percival J, Milner D, Wallace-Bell M. *Tobacco Control and Smoking Cessation: the role of the nurse* Geneva: International Council of Nurses, 2003.

24 • McEwen A, Hajek P, McRobbie H, *et al. Manual of Smoking Cessation* Oxford: Blackwell Publishing, 2006.

25 • Twigg L, Moon G, Walker S. *The Smoking Epidemic in England* London: Health Development Agency, 2004.

26 • Royal College of Physicians. *Nicotine Addiction in Britain* London: Royal College of Physicians, 2000.

27 • Boffretta P, Pershagen G, Jockel K H, *et al.* Cigar and pipe smoking and lung cancer risk: a multi-centre study from Europe *Journal of National Cancer Institute* 1999; **91(8)**: 697–701.

28 • Chao A, Thun MJ, Henley S J, *et al.* Cigarette smoking, use of other tobacco products and stomach cancer mortality in US adults: the Cancer Prevention Study 11 *International Journal of Cancer* 2002; **101(4)**: 380–9.

29 • Action on Smoking and Health. *Essential Information 11: stopping smoking: the benefits and aids to quitting* London: ASH, 2007.

30 • Butler C C, Pill R, Stott N C. Qualitative study of patients' perceptions of doctors' advice to quit smoking: implications for opportunistic health promotion *British Medical Journal* 1998; **316(7148)**: 1878–81.

31 • Department of Health. *Giving Up for Life* London: DH, 2004, www.givingupsmoking. co.uk [accessed January 2009].

32 • Thistlethwaite J, Morris P. *The Patient–Doctor Consultation in Primary Care: theory and practice* London: RCGP, 2006.

33 • Heatherton T F, Koslowski L T, Frecker R C. The Fagerström tolerance questionnaire *British Journal of Addiction* 1991; **86(9)**: 1119–27.

34 • World Health Organization. *The World Partnership to Reduce Tobacco Dependence* Copenhagen: WHO, 2000.

35 • Rotter J B. Generalized expectancies for internal versus external control of reinforcement *Psychological Monographs* 1966; **80**: 1–28.

36 • Department of Health. *Stop Smoking Start Living* London: DH, 2007, http:// gosmokefree.nhs.uk/downloads/108281_main_guide_double.pdf [accessed January 2009].

37 • Office for National Statistics. *Living in Britain: the 2002 General Household Survey* London: ONS, 2004.

38 • Benowitz N, Jacob P, Kozlowski L, *et al.* Influence of smoking fewer cigarettes on exposure to tar, nicotine and carbon monoxide *New England Journal of Medicine* 1986; **315(21)**: 1310–13.

39 • West R, McEwan A. *Sex and Smoking: comparisons between male and female smokers* London: Action on Smoking and Health, 1999.

40 • Hackshaw A K, Law M R, Wald N J. The accumulated evidence of lung cancer and environmental tobacco smoke *British Medical Journal* 1997; **315**: 980–8.

41 • Law M R, Morris J K, Wald N J. Environmental tobacco smoke exposure and ischaemic heart disease: an evaluation of the evidence *British Medical Journal* 1997; **315**: 973–80.

42 • Anderson H R, Cook D G. Passive smoking and sudden infant death syndrome: review of the epidemiological evidence *Thorax* 1997; **52**: 1003–9.

Asthma

4

Stephen Holmes and Monica Fletcher

Chapter aims

This chapter considers the diagnosis, the management and the general impact of asthma on patients and society.

Learning outcomes

After reading this chapter you will have refreshed your knowledge of:

▷ the prevalence of asthma and its impact on NHS and practice workload
▷ the impact asthma has on people's lives
▷ how to make an effective diagnosis of asthma and when to refer
▷ appropriate treatment strategies for people with asthma.

Initial self-assessment

Before reading this chapter we suggest that you consider the following:

1 ▷ list the clinical features that would make you consider the diagnosis of asthma as a high probability
2 ▷ how would you differentiate clinically between chronic obstructive pulmonary disease (COPD) and asthma?
3 ▷ you are called to visit a 45-year-old woman with acute wheezing with a background of longstanding asthma. List the key clinical features and likely management strategies you would use to care for her. What would make you consider hospital admission?
4 ▷ what areas would you cover in an 'asthma review'?

After reading the chapter you might wish to revisit your answers.

Overview

Asthma is a common condition that affects people of all ages. It can be controlled but many of our patients suffer significant disability for a variety of reasons. Asthma can result in absence from work, hospitalisation and death. It is a significant part of general practice workload. The evidence would suggest that the burden of the disease on our patients can be reduced by effective primary health care and high-quality management using appropriate self-help and pharmacological interventions.

Workload for the average general practitioner

The average general practitioner (GP) with 2000 patients will have around 120 people with asthma; they will consult on average three times a year for their asthma and will be seen on average six times a year.[1-4] The prevalence has not changed a great deal over time; current prevalence is estimated by the Quality and Outcomes Framework (QOF) data[5,6] at 5.7 per cent across England. This equates to a practice of 10,000 patients having 570 people with asthma.

Definition

Although there are several different definitions of asthma, all the definitions now contain common themes. The Global Initiative for Asthma (GINA) guidelines definition of asthma is:

a chronic inflammatory disorder of the airways in which many cells and cellular elements play a role. The chronic inflammation is associated with airway hyper-responsiveness that leads to recurrent episodes of wheezing, breathlessness, chest tightness and coughing, particularly at night or in the early morning. These episodes are usually associated with widespread, but variable, airflow obstruction within the lung that is often reversible either spontaneously or with treatment.[7]

The airways inflammation produces four forms of airway limitation:

▷ acute bronchoconstriction
▷ swelling of the airway wall
▷ chronic mucous plug formation
▷ airway wall remodelling.

From a clinical and primary care perspective it is important to remember that asthma:

▷ is an inflammatory disease (inhaled corticosteroids reduce this inflammation)
▷ can be triggered by a wide range of stimuli (but most are not identified clinically)
▷ is a variable condition with intermittent symptoms and signs (symptoms and signs are often absent in patients attending the surgery)
▷ can vary widely in severity, clinical course and response to treatment.

Prevalence and epidemiological factors

The exact prevalence of asthma across a population is difficult to ascertain. This is due to the variability of asthma and also to changes in both diagnostic criteria and the patient's perceptions of his or her symptoms.

In the UK there are varying estimates of prevalence. Research from Asthma UK suggests that around 5.2 million people in the UK suffer from asthma,[1-4] of which 1 million are children under 16 years. This equates to around 9.2 per cent of the population. Recent data from the National Health Service Primary Care QOF suggest the prevalence of asthma, in people over 8 years taking inhaled corticosteroids in England, is 5.8 per cent. The lowest prevalence in the UK is quoted as 4.5 per cent (in North Central London) and the highest prevalence 6.4 per cent (in Devon and Cornwall).[4] This might be linked to quality of the primary care disease registers rather than real prevalence. The QOF figure does not include the very significant number of patients who use their inhalers only irregularly and do not use inhaled corticosteroids.

Suffice it to say, asthma is very common, affects people often throughout their lives and is far more common than diabetes and coronary heart disease.

In adults there are more women with asthma (60:40) but in children this statistic is reversed.[8-11] Asthma is most commonly diagnosed in childhood or early adulthood but people can still develop the condition as they get older. Asthma is the single most common long-term condition in children. The diagnosis in children has varied over time in view of the perceived stigma associated with the condition and the perceived nature of presentation in children. This is covered in more detail in Chapter 6.

It is important to establish the work that people are doing if they develop asthma as an adult. Asthma is thought to be the commonest industrial disease in the developed world. It is estimated that 9–15 per cent of adult onset asthma is due to occupational causes.[12] Removal from the trigger at an early stage can prevent worsening asthma, hence in this group it is worthwhile considering specialist help.[13, 14]

There has been no clear difference found between different ethnic groups. However, in epidemiological studies the prevalence varies widely between different countries, being commonest in Australia, New Zealand, the UK and the USA. The prevalence appears to be lower in Indonesia, Romania, China and Russia.[15, 16]

Risk factors for developing asthma

The British Asthma Guidelines[14] highlight the following predisposing factors that increase the likelihood of development or persistence of asthma. These include:

▷ coexistence of atopic disease
▷ family history of atopic disease, especially maternal
▷ bronchiolitis in infancy
▷ male gender in pre-pubertal asthma – more commonly 'growing out' of asthma in the transition to adulthood
▷ female gender being a risk factor in asthma developing in the transition from childhood to adulthood
▷ age at presentation of wheeze (most who wheeze below the age of 2 years 'grow out' of the wheezing at 6–11 years), though a family history of atopy makes this less likely.

Making a diagnosis of asthma

The diagnosis of asthma can be primarily made on clinical grounds, though some tests and investigations are recommended to confirm the diagnosis, as is the documentation of a successful trial of treatment.

Potential presenting symptoms (these are frequently episodic) are:

▷ cough
▷ shortness of breath
▷ chest tightness
▷ wheezing.

These are often worse at night or after exertion.
There are sometimes triggers including:

▷ pollen
▷ house dust mite
▷ viral or bacterial infections
▷ exercise
▷ pets (often furry or feathered)
▷ cigarette smoke
▷ cold air
▷ irritant dusts or vapours
▷ atmospheric pollution
▷ stress
▷ foods
▷ occupational sensitisers (e.g. isocyanates, rubber)
▷ drugs (non-steroidal anti-inflammatory drugs, beta-blockers).

Additional history that might suggest the diagnosis of asthma is more likely includes:

▷ personal or family history of asthma or atopy
▷ history of worsening after aspirin or other drugs
▷ a recognised pattern to the symptoms (work or hobby linked).

There are some features which suggest that asthma is *less* likely, including:

▷ cough in the absence of wheeze or breathlessness
▷ prominent dizziness, light-headedness, peripheral tingling
▷ repeatedly normal clinical examination even when symptomatic
▷ no evidence of airway narrowing when symptomatic
▷ voice disturbance
▷ symptoms with colds only
▷ chronic productive cough
▷ significant smoking history (>20 pack years)
▷ cardiac disease.[14]

Examination

The examination of a patient presenting in general practice can be *entirely normal* when the patient is asymptomatic or has minimal symptoms. As the severity worsens examination findings are usually easier to detect. However, in severe cases some of the findings are again not detectable.

The key sign on examination that suggests a diagnosis of asthma is *a prolonged expiratory wheeze that is generalised, bilateral and polyphonic.*

Other factors in the examination help to determine the severity. These would include:

▷ general condition of patient
▷ signs of anxiety and fear
▷ colour (cyanosis)
▷ respiratory rate
▷ pulse rate and blood pressure
▷ 'silent chest'.

Investigations

Investigations in primary care are used either to help support the clinical diagnosis or exclude other conditions. The peak flow meter is readily available in primary care now and, increasingly, measurement of FEV_1 (forced expiratory volume in one second) is easy within a normal primary care consultation. Lung function testing equipment is present in most practices, if needed. The aim of investigations is to demonstrate reversible airway obstruction, and can be used in most people over the age of 7 years.

It is worthwhile considering a chest X-ray in patients who present atypically *or* if they are presenting with new symptoms. Asthma is very common – and can coexist with other conditions, for example pneumothorax or carcinoma.

Pulse oximetry is a useful method of checking oxygen saturation in the acute asthma episode, and again this investigation is much more readily available in primary care now.

Differential diagnosis

Clinically it is important to consider other conditions that might present with some similarities to asthma. These are listed in Box 4.1.

The three-part process for a strong diagnosis

Although in an acute situation (p. 56) when urgent management of the patient is required as a priority, it is often possible to make a diagnosis of asthma based on the following 'three parts':

1 ▷ good history compatible with asthma
2 ▷ objective evidence of airways variability
3 ▷ evidence of response to treatment.

Looking at these in more detail:

Box 4.1 ○ *Conditions with similarities to asthma*

▶ Chest infection/upper respiratory infection.

▶ COPD.

▶ Left ventricular failure ('cardiac asthma').

▶ Tumour (laryngeal, tracheal, lung).

▶ Bronchiectasis.

▶ Foreign body.

▶ Interstitial lung disease.

▶ Pulmonary emboli.

▶ Aspiration.

▶ Gastro-oesophageal reflux disease.

▶ Vocal cord dysfunction, post-tracheostomy stenosis.

▶ Psychological dyspnoea (panic attacks, anxiety states, hyperventilation syndrome).

▶ Pneumothorax.

Source: adapted from British Thoracic Society and Scottish Intercollegiate Guidelines Network.[14]

A good history compatible with asthma

This can be established at the consultation, and can cover the areas highlighted earlier. In general, we would be looking for a good history suggestive of asthma with, perhaps, some predisposing risks (atopy or family history). The BTS/SIGN guidelines make reference to the probability of asthma.[14] This is a helpful concept and is based on objective tests where possible, a good history and finally a trial of treatment.

Objective evidence of airways variability

This can be done, in accordance with British Asthma Guidelines, in several ways.

CLINICAL EXAMINATION/TESTS

Clinical examination can reveal prolonged expiratory wheeze with a reduced peak flow rate. When the patient is given a short-acting beta-agonist it would be expected that the wheeze improves or disappears and that there is an improvement in peak flow rate.

PEAK FLOW DIARY OVER TWO-WEEK PERIOD

Patients are provided with a peak flow meter (available on an NHS prescription). They are asked to measure a best peak flow twice a day (morning and evening) for a two-week period, looking for variability. This method was widely advocated in previous guidelines. However, clinicians often highlighted the difficulties that patients had in producing the charts or bringing them back for evaluation. Similarly, interpretation was often very difficult and the sensitivity and specificity is low in the research.[17] *Findings suggestive of asthma* would be 'a more than 20 per cent diurnal variation on at least 3 days in a week for two weeks'.[14] However, peak flow monitoring, although used at times for evaluation of treatment interventions or in occupational asthma, is no longer routinely recommended for diagnostic purposes.

LUNG FUNCTION TESTS

These are often performed in primary care, although their reliability in this environment has been questioned.[18] In general, however, with appropriate training in the technique, results can be reproducible.

Findings suggestive of asthma would be more than 15 per cent (and 200 ml) increase in FEV_1 after:

▷ **either** a short-acting beta$_2$-agonist (salbutamol 400 mcg by metered dose inhaler and spacer or 2.5 mg salbutamol by nebuliser)
▷ **or** after a trial of oral corticosteroids (e.g. prednisolone 30 mg per day for 14 days)
▷ **or** after a trial of 200 mcg twice-daily beclometasone by inhalation for 6–8 weeks.[14]

Evidence of response to treatment

Depending on the severity of symptoms initial treatment can be started with either oral or inhaled corticosteroids, in association with short-acting beta-agonists. In clinical practice it would be appropriate to assess at review both subjective and objective evidence of improvement of symptoms (both daytime and nocturnal).

Ideally the diagnosis would be made with good history and examination findings, objective lung function assessment and a good response to treatment. It is important to recognise that in primary care this is often made over a period of time.

Positive findings occur in around 70–80 per cent of untreated patients[20] and, although figures are less convincing in those already treated, it should be possible to diagnose the majority of patients in routine primary care practice.

Referral to specialist colleagues

The British Asthma Guidelines sensibly suggest referral to specialist colleagues when there is:

▷ an unclear diagnosis
▷ an unexpected clinical finding (*i.e. crackles, clubbing, cyanosis, cardiac disease*)
▷ unexplained restrictive spirometry
▷ a suspected occupational asthma
▷ persistent non-variable breathlessness
▷ a monophonic wheeze or stridor
▷ persistent chest pain
▷ prominent systemic features (*myalgia, fever, weight loss*)
▷ chronic sputum production
▷ CXR shadowing
▷ marked blood eosinophilia ($>1 \times 10^9/l$)

In addition, it would often be appropriate to refer to a specialist colleague when a patient determinedly requests this or when the clinician believes specialist input will consolidate primary care advice and facilitate better care.

When the diagnosis is not clear other investigations can be used to support the diagnosis in asthma. The following are usually performed in secondary care:

▷ exercise testing – lung function testing can be used to show a 15 per cent decrease in FEV_1 after exertion for six minutes
▷ methacholine challenge – lung function testing after administration of nebulised methacholine
▷ induced sputum eosinophil measurements
▷ fractional exhaled nitric oxide concentration (FENO).[19]

Management

A clear diagnosis of asthma is the cornerstone of good management. Once the diagnosis is made the clinician can set out to work with the patient to minimise symptoms, improve quality of life and reduce the impact of the disease on the patient's life.

The extent of control at present

In clinical trials it is possible to gain good control with current medication and good clinical support.[21] Despite these advantages there is still a great deal of work required to improve symptom control in people with asthma. Asthma UK[22] research suggests that in the UK 50 per cent of patients have severe asthma symptoms. This equates to 500,000 with difficult-to-control asthma and 2,100,000 with poorly controlled asthma. Current estimates from research elsewhere[23,24] would suggest that 70 per cent of people with asthma have regular symptoms relating to their condition. This situation does not appear to have improved over the last 15 years.[25]

The Royal College of Physicians' (RCP) three questions to improve the health of asthma patients[26] are often asked in primary care. These have been adapted to cover allergy and smoking with a more detailed questionnaire developed by the GPIAG and Allergy UK.[27] This is especially useful as those who smoke are less likely to gain benefit from inhaled corticosteroids at low dose.[28] There are other useful validated questionnaires for use in primary care, including the Asthma Control Test (ACT) and the Asthma Control Questionnaire (ACQ), both of which are cited in the BTS/SIGN guidelines.[14]

Box 4.2 ○ **GPIAG/Allergy UK six-point asthma and allergic rhinitis questionnaire**

In the last week:

1 ▶ did asthma affect your lifestyle (sport, work, school)?

2 ▶ were you affected/woken up by asthma symptoms (including cough, wheeze, breathlessness)?

3 ▶ did you experience asthma symptoms (including cough, wheeze, breathlessness)?

4 ▶ did you have any of the following symptoms when not having a cold: itchy, runny, blocked nose, catarrh or sneezing?

5 ▶ have you required any steroid tablets for worsening asthma in the last year?

6 ▶ have you smoked in the last 36 hours?

Source: GPIAG.[27] Reproduced with permission from GPIAG/Allergy UK.

ASTHMA

Acute asthma and the risk of death

It is frightening to think that one in every 250 deaths worldwide is from asthma.[29] Although the death rate from asthma in the UK is less than many countries (mortality data)[30] this is still 1400 deaths per year.[31] This equates to an asthma death in the UK every 8 hours.

As many as 90 per cent of the deaths from asthma are preventable.[32-34]

The research clearly shows that in many situations when somebody dies from asthma: [14]

▷ the patient has chronically severe asthma
▷ many are not on adequate inhaled corticosteroids
▷ many have had referral to secondary care delayed and have inadequate acute management of their asthma (oral steroids/beta-agonists)
▷ many are not adequately followed up when significant risk factors can be identified (see below) and do not have self-management plans.

The risk factors for death from asthma can be divided into medical and behavioural/psycho-social; these are often present in combination.

Box 4.3 ○ *Medical risk for death from asthma*

▶ Previous near-fatal episode of asthma (i.e. previous ventilation or ICU admission at any stage).
▶ Previous hospital admission for asthma, especially within the last year.
▶ Repeated attendance for emergency care, especially within the last year.
▶ Requiring three or more asthma medications.
▶ High use of beta$_2$-agonists.
▶ 'Brittle asthma'.

Box 4.4 ○ *Behavioural and psycho-social risks of death from asthma*

▶ Non-compliance with treatment or monitoring.
▶ Failure to attend appointments or previous self-discharge from hospital.
▶ Psychiatric illness or learning difficulties.
▶ Misuse of alcohol or drugs.
▶ Current or recent major tranquilliser use.
▶ Income or employment problems, social isolation.
▶ Severe domestic, marital or legal stress, child abuse.

Management in primary care

In many healthcare communities the wider respiratory team is based on a cohort of trained respiratory nurses (in primary care widely supported by the National Respiratory Training Centre, now Education for Health), along with respiratory nurse specialists within the hospital environment and GPs supported by their specialist respiratory colleagues.

Practices have computerised disease registers and this has revolutionised the ability to identify, recall and assess the care provided in primary care. More recently, this has been strengthened by the use of a QOF to promote quality parameters in chronic disease management.[35]

The management has been split into:

▷ the asthma review
▷ interventions for chronic asthma
▷ management of acute asthma.

The asthma review

In order to work effectively with patients to minimise symptoms from their asthma it is vital to ensure that asthma reviews fulfil a number of parameters.

The review should:

1 ▷ be convenient to the patient and the professional
2 ▷ provide an opportunity for shared understanding and agreed management strategies to manage his or her condition
3 ▷ facilitate data collection (for assuring quality of care).

In a good-quality asthma review it would be important to:

1 ▷ assess quality of *control* (typically using the RCP's three questions, or the adapted GPIAG / Allergy UK six questions)
2 ▷ *understand* patient and family views on asthma care (ideas, concerns and expectations) and map these to realistic targets
3 ▷ review lung function (*peak flow* reading)
4 ▷ review the use of *medications* and ability to use inhaler
5 ▷ review coexisting and *associated problems* (medical and psycho-social) – smoking cessation, obesity, potential pregnancy, work changes, allergic rhinitis
6 ▷ review a *personalised asthma action plan* with the patient that is geared to his or her understanding, lifestyle and clinical condition.

Personalised asthma action plans in combination with self-management education are a proven way of improving health outcomes in those with asthma.[36] However, less than one in four patients have a plan at the current time.[31] These plans are well proven with structured education programmes and in secondary care patients who have been admitted, but less certain in general clinical practice in primary care. Despite this, providing the patient with personalised information about his or her condition and the best ways to manage it has immense face validity. It is difficult to understand how people are not able to manage their illness better when they know more about it!

A variety of 'template' plans are produced by organisations (including Asthma UK). However, the personalised plan needs to be individualised by a skilled clinician in consultation with the patient.

Figure 4.1 ○ *Asthma Action Plan*

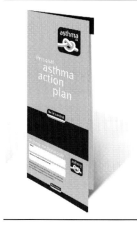

Source: image reproduced with permission from Asthma UK.

Within primary care consultations there are computerised templates that facilitate data collection and structured clinical care within the NHS.[37]

New modalities

It should be noted that if a patient has his or her own peak flow meter an entire review could be reasonably carried out by telephone (apart from the assessment of inhaler use); research has shown[38] that this can be as effective as face-to-face review. Traditionally, most reviews are carried out face to face, though the failure-to-attend rate has been an issue in primary care – hence more clinicians and patients are happy with telephone consultation.

Modern technology with computers, mobile phones and texting is creating opportunities for patients to obtain advice from a much wider range of sources than was previously possible.

Coexisting disease – allergic rhinitis

There is considerable evidence of the link between asthma and allergic rhinitis (AR) or rhinosinusitis (clinically, pathologically, anatomically and epidemiologically).[39] Similarly, there is good evidence that people with poorly controlled asthma gain improved symptom control if their allergic rhinitis is controlled.[40] Similarly, people with allergic rhinitis whose condition is not well controlled should have a coexistent diagnosis of asthma considered and, if present, should be managed in combination. This is covered in more detail in Chapter 5.

Non-pharmacological

As asthma is a very common condition worldwide, not unexpectedly there are many suggested treatments available with varying degrees of medical and non-medical support.[14] For many people the non-pharmacological options provide a more desirable way of trying to ease asthma symptoms. There are some situations where this approach should be commended and supported strongly, where the scientific evidence is robust. There are many non-pharmacological interventions where there is little, no or even some evidence to suggest harm.[14]

There are no reliable primary prevention methods for asthma at the current time.

Table 4.1 ○ *Primary prevention*

Allergen avoidance	No evidence for primary prevention
Breastfeeding	Mixed evidence.[41] Appears to reduce early wheeze, might increase asthma in children over six years
Dietary changes	No evidence except for limited epidemiological data on fish oil consumption in childhood reducing prevalence of asthma
Avoiding pollutants	Limited evidence

Smoking	No evidence that smoking exposure changes the likelihood of developing asthma. Significant evidence that smoking increases early childhood wheeze and other respiratory-related conditions

Table 4.2 ○ **Secondary prevention**

Allergen avoidance	No strong evidence
House dust mite avoidance	No cost-effective interventions proven[42] but in parents with commitment it is reasonable to recommend
Pets	There is no evidence in trials that pet removal results in improved asthma control. There are still, however, a considerable number of experts who through their clinical experience recommend pet removal for patients

House dust mite avoidance

House dust mite avoidance[42,43] is very difficult to achieve in practice and is not felt to be cost-effective. Despite this, from parents' experience and advertising many are often keen to try. If this is the case the following are recommended:

▷ complete barrier bed covering systems
▷ removal of carpets
▷ removal of soft toys from bed
▷ high-temperature washing of bed linen
▷ acaricides to soft furnishings
▷ dehumidification.

Smoking

Smoking appears to reduce the efficacy of inhaled corticosteroids[28] and increase bronchial hyperreactivity.[45]

Patients and their family and friends who smoke should be offered help in giving up (see Chapter 3). In addition to problems with asthma there are widely recognised problems linked to smoking, including other respiratory diseases, cardiovascular disease and cancers. Giving up smoking has been shown to improve asthma symptoms[46] as well as reduce risks of other conditions.

Complementary therapy

Considerable research and many recommendations are made but as yet there is little convincing evidence to help to recommend these options.

Table 4.3 ○ *Efficacy of complementary therapies*

Acupuncture	Not beneficial[47]
Air ionisers	Potential harm, no benefit[43]
Family therapy	Two small trials suggest some benefit[48]
Herbal/traditional Chinese medicine	Not beneficial – conclusion from analysis of 17 trials[49]
Homeopathy	Insufficient evidence[50]
Physical exercise	No improvement in lung function, but improved work capacity and general cardiopulmonary fitness[51]
Physical therapy (massage/chiropractor)	Not beneficial (chiropractor); no evidence for massage[52]

Pharmacological management of asthma

The management of asthma should be designed to control symptoms and disease process, whilst maintaining the patient on the lowest dose of safe medication. There is sometimes a balance that is required between these aims.

It is recommended that clinicians refer to the current British Asthma Guidelines (available on www.sign.ac.uk) and the *British National Formulary* as well as the Summary of Product Characteristics for detailed prescribing advice and information on medications used.

Control of symptoms can be defined as:

▷ minimal symptoms during the day and night
▷ no exacerbations
▷ minimal need for reliever therapy
▷ no limitation of exercise
▷ normal lung function.[14]

Asthma is an inflammatory condition that usually responds well to inhaled corticosteroids. Asthma is variable in its symptoms and severity. Over time the amount of medication required to control asthma might rise or fall.

Inhaler devices

The management of asthma (and COPD) is made more complex than many conditions pharmacologically, as many of the medications used are inhaled rather than ingested. This has resulted in a need to understand the rationale behind how a medication can be inhaled into the airways successfully and directly onto inflamed areas of lung, without the more systemic effects of treatments being noted elsewhere. This means that in asthma (and COPD) careful choice of an appropriate inhaler device is vital to good-quality care.

Key factors that should influence the choice of inhaler device a person with asthma uses are:

▷ safety
▷ efficacy
▷ cost
▷ patient's ability to use
▷ patient's preference.

There is a variety of inhaler devices available. Effectively they are either pressured metered dose inhaler (pMDI) or dry powder inhaler (DPI); of these some are breath actuated, while others require the patient to co-ordinate hand movement and breathing or use a further device (spacer).

There is considerable research at a scientific level into particle deposition in the lung and the relationship with particle size. The National Institute for Health and Clinical Excellence (NICE) technology appraisal[53] suggests that, if all things are equal, the most cost-effective preparation should be used. In most situations when patients have a choice, all things are not equal. In the past it was possible to obtain CFC-containing inhalers but, in line with the Montreal Protocol, these are being phased out.

The five most commonly used inhalers at the current time for people with asthma are:

▷ pMDI (salbutamol / terbutaline / formoterol / salmeterol / beclometasone dipropionate/ budesonide / ciclesonide/mometasone/fluticasone)
▷ pMDI and spacer (as above)
▷ breath actuated (as above)
▷ turbohaler device (budesonide / terbutaline/formoterol only)
▷ accuhaler (salbutamol / salmeterol / fluticasone).

Figure 4.2 ○ *Inhalers*

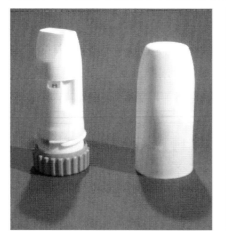
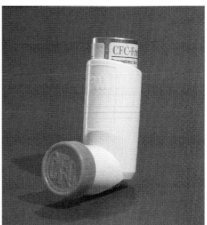
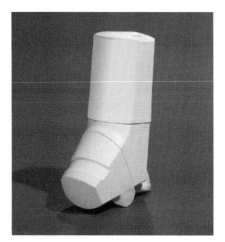
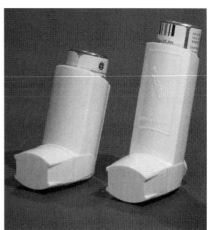
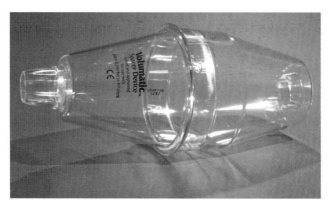

Source: reproduced by kind permission of Education for Health.

Stepwise treatment

A stepwise approach to management is advocated in asthma.[14] If control is poor (assuming a clinician reconsiders the diagnosis, symptoms and checks on use of medications) then treatment needs to be stepped up. If control is achieved for a period of time it is often worthwhile reducing treatment levels to the minimum that control symptoms.

Step 1 – mild intermittent asthma

In mild intermittent asthma use of a short-acting bronchodilator is recommended. This, in general, is a short-acting beta-agonist (as speed of onset of action and side effect profile is better). There are two widely used short-acting bronchodilators (salbutamol and terbutaline), both of which are available in a variety of inhaler devices.

Step 2 – regular preventer therapy

If a short-acting bronchodilator is required for more than 3 days in a week or the patient wakes at night, it is likely that there is chronic inflammation present and low-dose inhaled corticosteroids are recommended. Most people are controlled on 400 mcg (i.e. 200 mcg b.d.) of beclometasone dipropionate (BDP – CFC containing) in adults or 200 mcg in children. There is a variety of other inhaled corticosteroids available and a comparable dose should be calculated.

At levels of 800 mcg of BDP in adults and 400 mcg in children there is no evidence of systemic side effects. Above this dose there are more systemic side effects. It is important to inform and discuss steroid safety and use with patients and carers as this is a common area of concern. The dose of inhaled steroid should not be increased above 800 mcg (400 mcg in children) unless add-on therapy has been considered and possibly tried.

When caring for people with asthma it is as important, if symptom control is poor, to evaluate shared understanding, concordance and inhaler technique issues, as well as considering potential causes other than asthma for the symptoms, as it is to step-up therapy.

Step 3 – add-on therapy

First-choice add-on therapy in those over 6 years old is a long-acting bronchodilator (formoterol, salmeterol) in addition to the inhaled corticosteroid.

This has been shown to reduce exacerbations and improve both lung function and patient symptoms.[54,55]

If regular dosing is not controlling symptoms then a single maintenance and reliever therapy (SMART) can be considered prior to addition of other medications.[56-61] This is using formoterol and budesonide in combination in a regular twice-daily regime and as needed.

If this is unsuccessful then the following preparations should be considered and possibly tried (but discontinued if no effect).

CHROMONES

These are effective in some children between the ages of 5–12 years and have some effect in adults. In current clinical practice, however, these are now rarely used.

LEUKOTRIENE RECEPTOR ANTAGONISTS

These have some anti-inflammatory effects and are a useful potential addition in adults. Leukotriene receptor antagonists (LTRA) are used more frequently in children and have some effect in allergic rhinitis as well as asthma.

THEOPHYLLINES

These have shown some anti-inflammatory effect but side effects are common and monitoring is needed.

ORAL LONG-ACTING BRONCHODILATORS

These can improve lung function and symptoms but side effects are common.

Step 4 – addition of fourth drug

If control is poor on short-acting beta-agonist, higher-dose inhaled corticosteroid plus inhaled long-acting beta-agonist, then the addition of the following might help to control symptoms:

▷ LTRA
▷ theophylline
▷ long-acting beta-agonist tablets

or increase of inhaled corticosteroid to 2000 mcg per day BDP or equivalent.

Step 5 – continuous or frequent use of oral steroids

With children and many adults, before proceeding to step 5, specialist referral should be strongly considered to review the diagnosis and therapeutic
options. For patients in this category the following should be considered:

▷ regular blood pressure monitoring
▷ monitoring of bone mineral density
▷ monitoring of blood glucose
▷ monitoring for cataract and raised intraocular pressure.

Other medications described at step 5 should be initiated and monitored
in collaboration with specialist care. These include: methotrexate, gold, oral
cyclosporin and omalizumab (anti-IgE).

Special situations

There are some situations where management can be more complex and
specialised. For adults who develop asthma for the first time alternative
diagnoses and occupational causes should be strongly considered. Children
require special consideration as the diagnosis is often harder to make – and
high-dose treatment can adversely affect growth. Pregnancy is also a common area where confusion can occur. There are other causes of breathlessness linked in with pregnancy – including physiological causes linked
to rib splaying and increased progestogen levels, pulmonary embolus and
anaemia, as well as a varied response to treatments and concerns around
the use of medications and their safety. Similarly, other medical conditions
can make treatments more complex, and high-risk patients who have had
serious respiratory problems in the past can complicate the typical picture
of asthma.

In general, exercise-induced asthma is often linked with symptoms at
night and in other situations, indicating increased treatment is required.
However, for elite athletes and more complex cases, special testing and considerations should be made.

What does this tell us? The majority of our patients can be well controlled in primary care where a generalist is managing a commonly occurring
problem. However, we are lucky to have support from specialists who deal
with special situations and more complex asthma, and we should be com-
fortable asking for their help and advice when needed.

Management of acute asthma

Patients with acute asthma [14] can present to a wide number of healthcare professionals and we are aware that early and appropriate treatment can reduce the severity of the episode and reduce mortality.

Clinically it is important to assess the patient appropriately.

Life-threatening asthma is recognised by the following features (note: not all have to be present and a previous history of life-threatening asthma should flag up caution):

▷ peak flow rate of less than 33 per cent of best or predicted
▷ pulse oximetry reading of less than 92 per cent
▷ cyanosis
▷ silent chest
▷ poor respiratory effort
▷ bradycardia
▷ hypotension
▷ confusion
▷ coma
▷ exhaustion.

Acute severe asthma is recognised by: a peak flow of 33–50 per cent of best or predicted; respiratory rate of more than 25/m; heart rate of more than 110/m; and an inability to complete sentences.

Moderate exacerbations of asthma are recognised by a peak flow of 50–75 per cent of best or predicted with no features of acute severe asthma.

Those with life-threatening asthma should be transferred to hospital as soon as possible, as should those with symptoms of acute severe asthma persisting after initial treatment. Those who, after initial treatment, achieve a peak flow of more than 75 per cent of normal can in general be treated in the community, unless there are specific risks in the patient's previous history.

Treatments for acute asthma include:

1 ▷ oxygen (high flow rate if available)
2 ▷ short-acting bronchodilator (preferably through an oxygen-driven nebuliser) or, if this is not available and the condition less severe, via nebuliser or large-volume spacer device
3 ▷ steroid therapy (this is usually 40–50 mg of prednisolone orally once daily for at least five days or recovery for 72 hours)

4 ▷ in acute or life-threatening asthma ipratropium bromide can be added as a nebulised solution

5 ▷ other treatments (magnesium sulphate; IV theophyllines) should only be used with the advice and supervision of senior medical staff.

Some of these treatments will be available in primary care. There is strong evidence, including a Cochrane review, to demonstrate that the use of large-volume spacers in moderate to severe asthma is equally efficacious to nebulisers. Every practice should have one available with an MDI for administration in an emergency

It is good practice to ensure that any patients who have required hospital admission or oral steroid use for an acute asthma attack are carefully reviewed following this, and that plans are made to support their self-management with a personalised asthma action plan and tailored clinical supervision.

Conclusion

Asthma is a common long-term condition affecting a large number of people. There is a considerable amount we can do to help our patients with a careful diagnosis and balanced therapeutic interventions supported by education and personalised action plans. Although there is considerable mortality and morbidity from this condition, good-quality primary care can make a significant difference in both areas.

Further sources of information

General Practice Airways Group • **www.gpiag.org**.
British Thoracic Society • **www.brit-thoracic.org.uk**.
Scottish Intercollegiate Guidelines Network • **www.sign.ac.uk**.

References

1 • Department of Health. *Health Survey for England 2001* London: The Stationery Office, 2003.

2 • Bromley C, Sproston K, Shelton N. *Scottish Health Survey 2003* Edinburgh: The Stationery Office, 2005.

3 • Shaw A, McMunn A, Field J. *Scottish Health Survey 1998* Edinburgh: The Stationery Office, 2000.

4 • Office for National Statistics. *Census 2001* Newport: ONS, 2001.

5 • The Health and Social Care Information Centre. *National Quality and Outcomes Framework Statistics for England 2007/08*, www.ic.nhs.uk/qof [accessed January 2009].

6 • Ross Anderson H. Prevalence of asthma: is no longer increasing in some countries, but the reasons for this are unclear *British Medical Journal* 2005; **330**: 1037–8.

7 • Global Initiative for Asthma. *Global Strategy for Asthma Management and Prevention* 2007, www.ginasthma.org [accessed January 2009].

8 • Nicolai T, Pereszlenyiova-Bliznakova L, Illi S, *et al.* Longitudinal follow-up of the changing gender ratio in asthma from childhood to adulthood: role of delayed manifestation in girls *Pediatric Allergy and Immunology* 2003; **14**: 280–3.

9 • Health Survey for England. *Respiratory Symptoms, Atopic Conditions and Lung Function 2001*, www.archive2.official-documents.co.uk/document/deps/doh/survey01/rsac/rsac01.htm [accessed January 2009].

10 • de Marco R, Locatelli F, Sunyer J, *et al.* Differences in incidence of reported asthma related to age in men and women: a retrospective analysis of the data of the European Respiratory Health Survey *American Journal of Respiratory and Critical Care Medicine* 2000; **162**: 68–74.

11 • Eagan T M, Bakke P S, Eide G E, *et al.* Incidence of asthma and respiratory symptoms by sex, age and smoking in a community study *European Respiratory Journal* 2002; **19**: 599–605 (erratum, 2003; **21**: 735).

12 • British Occupational Health Research Foundation. *Occupational Asthma: identification, management and prevention* London: BOHRF, 2004.

13 • Health and Safety Executive, www.hse.gov.uk/asthma [accessed January 2009].

14 • British Thoracic Society and Scottish Intercollegiate Guidelines Network. British Guideline on the Management of Asthma *Thorax* 2008; **63**: 1–121, doi:10.1136/thx.2008.097741.

15 • ISAAC. Worldwide variations in the prevalence of asthma symptoms: the International Study of Asthma and Allergies in Childhood (ISAAC) *European Respiratory Journal* 1998; **12**: 315–35.

16 • Global Initiative for Asthma. *Global Strategy for Asthma Management and Prevention* GINA, 1995 (updated 2006), www.ginasthma.org/Guidelineitem.asp??l1=2&l2=1&intId=60 [accessed January 2009].

17 • Goldstein M F, Veza B A, Dunsky E H, *et al.* Comparisons of peak diurnal expiratory flow variation, postbronchodilator FEV_1 responses, and methacholine inhalation challenges in the evaluation of suspected asthma *Chest* 2001; **119**: 1010.

18 • Bolton C, Ionescu A, Edwards P, *et al.* Attaining a correct COPD diagnosis in general practice *Respiratory Medicine* 2005; **99**: 493–500.

19 • Berry M, Hargadon B, Morgan A, *et al.* Alveolar nitric oxide in adults with asthma *European Respiratory Journal* 2005; **25(6)**: 986–91.

20 • Gibson P G, Fujimura M, Niimi A. Eosinophilic bronchitis: clinical manifestations and implications for treatment *Thorax* 2002; **57(2)**: 178–82.

21 • Bateman E D, Boushey H A, Bousquet J, *et al.* Can guideline-defined asthma control be achieved? The Gaining Optimal Asthma ControL study *American Journal of Respiratory and Critical Care Medicine* 2004; **170**: 836–44.

22 • Asthma UK. *Living on a Knife Edge* London: Asthma UK, 2004.

23 • Haughney J, Barnes G, Partridge M, *et al.* The Living & Breathing Study: a study of patients' views of asthma and its treatment *Primary Care Respiratory Journal* 2004; **13**: 28–35.

24 • Partridge M R, van der Molen T, Myrseth S-E, *et al.* Attitudes and actions of asthma patients on regular maintenance therapy: the INSPIRE study *BMC Pulmonary Medicine* 2006; **6**: 13, www.biomedcentral.com/1471-2466/6/13 [accessed January 2009].

25 • Chinn S, Jarvis D, Burney P, *et al.* Increase in diagnosed asthma but not in symptoms in the European Community Respiratory Health Survey *Thorax* 2004; **59**: 646–51.

26 • Pearson M G, Bucknall C E (eds). *Measuring Clinical Outcome in Asthma: a patient focused approach* London: Royal College of Physicians, Clinical Effectiveness & Evaluation Unit, 1999.

27 • The 6 Point Asthma and Allergic Rhinitis Status Measure, www.gpiag.org/news/gp_diagnostic_tool.pdf [accessed January 2009].

28 • Thomson N C, Chaudhuri R, Livingston E. Asthma and cigarette smoking *European Respiratory Journal* 2004; **24**: 822–33.

29 • Rees J. Asthma control in adults *British Medical Journal* 2006; **332(7544)**: 767–71.

30 • Russell G. *Extent of Asthma in the UK* Lung and Asthma Information Agency, www.laia.ac.uk/asthma.htm [accessed January 2009].

31 • Asthma UK. *Where Do We Stand? Asthma in the UK today* London: Asthma UK, 2006, www.asthma.org.uk/all_about_asthma/publications/where_do_we.html [accessed January 2009].

32 • Wareham N J, Harrison B D, Jenkins P F, *et al.* A district confidential enquiry into deaths due to asthma *Thorax* 1993; **48**: 1117–20.

33 • Harrison B, Stephenson P, Mohan G, *et al.* An ongoing confidential enquiry into asthma deaths in the Eastern Region of the UK, 2001–2003 *Primary Care Respiratory Journal* 2004; **14**: 303–13.

34 • Anon. *PCG Cash Limits Mean Asthma Remains a Neglected Disease* Primary Care Report, 2000.

35 • GP Committee of the British Medical Association and the NHS Confederation. *Revisions to the GMS Contract, 2006/07: delivering investment in general practice* London: BMA and NHS Confederation, 2006, www.bma.org.uk/ap.nsf/Content/revisionnGMSFeb20062 [accessed January 2009].

36 • Gibson P G, Powell H. Written action plans for asthma: an evidence-based review of the key components *Thorax* 2004; **59(2)**: 94–9.

37 • NHS Confederation and the British Medical Association. *New GMS Contract* London: DH, 2005, www.dh.gov.uk [accessed January 2009].

38 • Pinnock H, Bawden R, Proctor S, *et al.* Accessibility, acceptability, and effectiveness in primary care of routine telephone review of asthma: pragmatic, randomised controlled trial *British Medical Journal* 2003; **326**: 477.

39 • Allergic Rhinitis and Its Impact on Asthma. *Management of Allergic Rhinitis and Its Impact on Asthma: a pocket guide for physicians and nurses* ARIA, 2001, www.whiar.org [accessed January 2009].

40 • Taramarcaz P, Gibson PG. Intranasal corticosteroids for asthma control in people with coexisting asthma and rhinitis *Cochrane Database of Systematic Reviews* 2003, Issue 4. Art. No.: CD003570. DOI: 10.1002/14651858.CD003570.

41 • Ram FSF, Ducharme FM, Scarlett J. Cow's milk protein avoidance and development of childhood wheeze in children with a family history of atopy *Cochrane Database of Systematic Reviews* 2007, Issue 2, Art. No.: CD003795. DOI: 10.1002/14651858. CD003795.pub2.

42 • Gøtzsche PC, Johansen HK, Schmidt LM, *et al*. House dust mite control measures for asthma *Cochrane Database of Systematic Reviews* 1998, Issue 3, Art. No.: CD001187.

43 • Warner JA, Marchant JL, Warner JO. Double blind trial of ionisers in children with asthma sensitive to the house dust mite *Thorax* 1993; **48(4)**: 330–3.

44 • Thomson NC, Chaudhuri R, Livingston E. Asthma and cigarette smoking *European Respiratory Journal* 2004; **24(5)**: 822–33.

45 • Tomlinson JEM, McMahon AD, Chaudhuri R, *et al*. Efficacy of low and high dose inhaled corticosteroid in smokers versus non-smokers with mild asthma *Thorax* 2005; **60(4)**: 282–7.

46 • Eisner M, Yelin EH, Henke J. Environmental tobacco smoke and adult asthma *American Journal of Respiratory and Critical Care Medicine* 1998; **158**: 170–5.

47 • McCarney RW, Brinkhaus B, Lasserson TJ, *et al*. Acupuncture for chronic asthma *Cochrane Database of Systematic Reviews* 2003, Issue 1, Art. No.: CD000008. DOI: 10.1002/14651858.CD000008.pub2.

48 • Yorke J, Shuldham C. Family therapy for asthma in children *Cochrane Database of Systematic Reviews* 1996, Issue 3, Art. No.: CD000089. DOI: 10.1002/14651858.CD000089. pub2.

49 • Arnold E, Clark CE, Lasserson TJ, *et al*. Herbal interventions for chronic asthma in adults and children *Cochrane Database of Systematic Reviews* 2008, Issue 1, Art. No.: CD005989. DOI: 10.1002/14651858.CD005989.pub2.

50 • McCarney RW, Linde K, Lasserson TJ. Homeopathy for chronic asthma *Cochrane Database of Systematic Reviews* 2003, Issue 3, Art. No.: CD000353. DOI: 10.1002/14651858. CD000353.pub2.

51 • Ram FSF, Robinson SM, Black PN, *et al*. Physical training for asthma *Cochrane Database of Systematic Reviews* 2005, Issue 3, Art. No.: CD001116. DOI: 10.1002/14651858. CD001116.pub2.

52 • Dennis J, Cates CJ. Alexander technique for chronic asthma *Cochrane Database of Systematic Reviews* 2000, Issue 2, Art. No.: CD000995. DOI: 10.1002/14651858.CD000995.

53 • National Institute for Health and Clinical Excellence. *Inhaler Devices for Routine Treatment of Chronic Asthma in Older Children (Aged 5–15 Years)* (Technology Appraisal Guidance No. 38) London: NICE, 2002.

54 • Ni Chroinin M, Greenstone IR, Danish A. *et al*. Long-acting beta$_2$-agonists versus placebo in addition to inhaled corticosteroids in children and adults with chronic asthma *Cochrane Database of Systematic Reviews* 2005, Issue 4, Art. No.: CD005535. DOI: 10.1002/14651858.CD005535.

55 • O'Byrne PM, Barnes PJ, Rodriguez-Roisin R, *et al*. Low dose inhaled budesonide and formoterol in mild persistent asthma: the OPTIMA randomized trial *American Journal of Respiratory and Critical Care Medicine* 2001; **164(8 Pt 1)**: 1392–7.

56 • National Prescribing Service. Budesonide with eformoterol dry powder inhaler (Symbicort) maintenance and reliever regimen for asthma *NPS RADAR* 2007, http:// nps.org.au/health_professionals/publications/nps_radar/issues/current/august_2007/ budesonide_with_eformoterol [accessed January 2009].

57 • Kuna P, Peters M J, Manjra A I, *et al.* Effect of budesonide/formoterol maintenance and reliever therapy on asthma exacerbations *International Journal of Clinical Practice* 2007; **61(5)**: 725–36.

58 • O'Byrne P M, Bisgaard H, Godard P P, *et al.* Budesonide/formoterol combination therapy as both maintenance and reliever medication in asthma *American Journal of Respiratory and Critical Care Medicine* 2005; **171**: 129–36.

59 • Rabe K F, Pizzichini E, Stallberg B, *et al.* Budesonide/formoterol in a single inhaler for maintenance and relief in mild-to-moderate asthma: a randomized, double-blind trial *Chest* 2006; **129**: 246–56.

60 • Vogelmeier C, D'Urzo A, Pauwels R, *et al.* Budesonide/formoterol maintenance and reliever therapy: an effective asthma treatment option? *European Respiratory Journal* 2005; **26**: 819–28.

61 • Rabe K F, Atienza T, Magyar P, *et al.* Effect of budesonide in combination with formoterol for reliever therapy in asthma exacerbations: a randomised controlled, double-blind study *Lancet* 2006; **368**: 744–53.

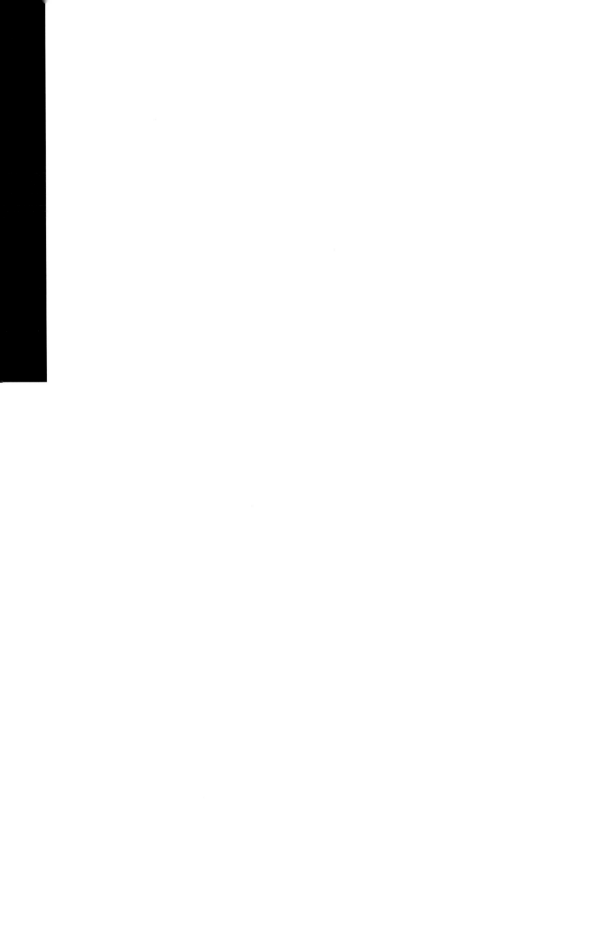

Allergy and allergic rhinitis

5

Samantha Walker and Aziz Sheikh

Chapter aims

This chapter will explore the definition and mechanisms of allergy, considering diagnosis and management, particularly focusing on allergic rhinitis.

Learning outcomes

After reading this chapter you will have considered:

▷ the definition and mechanisms of allergy
▷ how to make a diagnosis of allergy
▷ objective allergen testing
▷ the diagnosis and management of allergic rhinitis
▷ the management of anaphylaxis.

Initial self-assessment

For each of the following case examples consider what the differential diagnosis might be. What is the patient's/parent's agenda? How might you investigate/manage the patient?

1 ▷ Sukhi, a 5-year-old girl, is brought to you by her mother. She gets a generalised itchy rash after eating oranges. She is otherwise well, with no history of atopy.

2 ▷ George, a 14-year-old boy, is brought by his mother complaining of excessive flatulence and abdominal pain. She suggests that this has lessened since she changed him to dairy-free milk. He is overweight but otherwise well.

3 ▷ Pearline, a 37-year-old woman, gets swollen lips after eating takeaway meals. She is no more specific and denies any other problems.

Allergy and allergens

The term allergy was coined by the Austrian paediatrician Clemens von Pirquet in 1906 whilst working at Johns Hopkins Hospital in Baltimore.[1] Transmitted through German ('*allergie*'), it is etymologically derived from a conjunction of the Greek term '*allos*', meaning 'a deviation from the original state', and '*ergos*', meaning 'work' or 'action'.[2,3] Von Pirquet was therefore using the term to describe a generalised state of 'changed reactivity' following exposure to an antigen, which he defined as 'a foreign substance which by one or more applications stimulates the organism to a change in reaction'.[1] This changed reactivity thus encompassed the entire science of immunology including both immunity (protective) and hypersensitivity (harmful) states. The antigen could be either an infectious agent or an allergen.

More recently, the term allergy has frequently been limited to referring to immunoglobulin-E (IgE)-mediated hypersensitivity reactions only.[4] Allergy and hypersensitivity are thereby used as synonyms to describe any exaggerated response of the immune system to allergenic agents. Allergology as understood and practised in the UK is concerned in the main with IgE-mediated hypersensitivity reactions to allergenic antigens such as atopic eczema, food allergy, allergic rhinitis, asthma and anaphylaxis.[5] The term allergy however remains contested, with some academics arguing for the need to return to von Pirquet's original broader meaning.[5,6] The practice of many allergists is similarly somewhat incongruous, with many also caring for patients with a variety of conditions that often do not have an IgE-mediated pathophysiology, such as urticaria, difficult asthma in adults and non-allergic rhinitis.

An allergen is a foreign protein or hapten that has the ability to provoke formation of specific IgE antibodies, which may in turn result in an allergic response. A hapten is a small molecule that although, in itself, is incapable of inducing an antibody response, may do so when bound to a protein carrier. Common allergens encountered in the UK include aero-allergens (e.g. house dust mite, tree and grass pollens, and pet dander), food (e.g. cow's milk protein, eggs and peanuts) and the venom of stinging insects (e.g. from wasps and bees).

Mechanisms of allergy

Allergic reactions (e.g. the sneezing, itching and watery rhinorrhea seen in summer hay fever; the immediate generalised rash (urticaria) and subsequent anaphylaxis observed in severe peanut allergy) are classic examples of Type 1 hypersensitivity, first described by Gell and Coombs in 1963 (see Table 5.1).[7] They described an interaction between allergen (e.g. grass pollen, peanut) and mast cells. Mast cells are ubiquitous in the peripheral blood and tissues, and contain granules that in turn contain histamine. This is a potent chemical that causes itching due to irritation of nerve endings, redness due to vasodilatation of blood vessels, and swelling due to increased vascular permeability. This is via an antibody, subsequently named IgE.

Table 5.1 ○ *Immunological mechanisms of allergy*

Type	Principal effector	Example
	IgE	Anaphylaxis,* urticaria,* angioedema,* bronchospasm*
Type II – cytotoxic	IgG	Cytopenia, vasculitis
Type III – immune complex mediated	IgG	Serum sickness, vasculitis
Type IV – T-cell mediated	T-cell	Contact dermatitis, maculopapular rash, bullous (blistering) rashes

* These might also occur due to non-specific mechanisms.
Source: based on Gell and Coombs's classification of hypersensitivity reactions.[7,8]

The inhalation (via the nose or mouth), ingestion or injection of allergen results in a classic sequence of events: the allergen quickly forms a bridge between two allergen-specific IgE antibody molecules and mast cells, which then degranulate and release their contents. This leads to both the immediate release and new synthesis of the inflammatory chemicals (e.g. histamine, leukotrienes, prostaglandins, heparin and platelet-activating factor (PAF)) that produce the symptoms of an allergic reaction. IgE-mediated reactions can cause a spectrum of symptoms including flushing, itch, sneezing, nettle rash, wheeze, stridor, dizziness and loss of consciousness. The classic signs of allergy – itching, redness and swelling – and its classic time course – immediate symptoms, usually occurring within 15 minutes of exposure – mark the cornerstone of allergy diagnosis, and, at a simplistic level, allow the differentiation between allergic and non-allergic symptoms.

Definitions

'Atopy' is described as a hereditary predisposition to develop allergic symptoms and is defined clinically as a positive skin prick test or specific IgE blood test to one or more common aero-allergens. The term 'allergy' was first used in 1906[1] to describe 'altered reactivity' to substances in our environment. The term is currently used to describe an immunological response to common aero-allergens or food/drug allergens. This defines allergy as being quite separate from 'intolerance', an example of which includes migraine, which is seen in response to some foods. It is important to remember that atopic patients might not have symptoms on exposure to the allergen they test positive to, and so a diagnosis of allergy can not be made by the results of a skin or blood test alone.

Allergy diagnosis

Accurate allergy diagnosis depends on the concordance (or lack of it) between the history and the results of an objective measurement of allergen-specific IgE antibodies. Accurate history taking is of primary importance in establishing the role of allergy, and it is important to question patients closely. Particular questions to ask include the following.

▷ Do the symptoms seem to fit the pattern of histamine release, i.e. do symptoms include redness, itching or swelling? It is important to look out for the manifestation of histamine release in different organ systems; for example, histamine-induced nerve irritation manifests in the nose as sneezing, in the skin as itching and in the lungs as wheezing; increased vascular permeability manifests in the skin as a wheal similar in appearance to a nettle rash, in the nose as nasal blockage and systemically as hypotension (due to sudden and excessive leakage from major vessels).

▷ What is the relationship between allergen exposure and symptoms? As mentioned previously, typical IgE-mediated allergic symptoms occur within approximately 15 minutes of allergen exposure. This is helpful to remember when trying to interpret a history of possible food-related symptoms. An early sign of food-related anaphylaxis is a histamine-induced generalised itchy rash occurring immediately after the ingestion of a food; abdominal pain, flatulence and general malaise (with no sign of itching, redness or swelling) occurring 6–8 hours after a meal are more likely to be the result of a food intolerance.

▷ Is there more than one organ system involved? Because mast cells are present at many different sites throughout the body, IgE-mediated allergy tends to occur in more than one organ system. Thus a patient who wheezes when near a cat is also likely to develop a runny nose and sneezing. A rash attributed to penicillin is more likely to be IgE-mediated if it is accompanied by symptoms in other organ systems such as wheezing, vomiting or diarrhoea. Allergy is a systemic disease, and thus patients are likely to present with symptoms in more than one organ system during their lifetimes. Babies who have food-related eczema often have asthma as a child and then hay fever as an adolescent, and it is important to be on the look-out for new manifestations of allergic symptoms in subsequent consultations.

▷ Is there an obvious allergic trigger? In a situation where the history points to an obvious allergic trigger, an objective test of specific IgE might not be necessary. In patients where the relationship between exposure and symptoms is unclear, a skin prick test or blood test might be helpful, although it is important to remember that evidence of specific IgE does not imply causality. Allergen avoidance underpins both the asthma and rhinitis management guidelines, advice which cannot be given with any confidence unless a causal relationship is established.

▷ Is there a past history of allergic disease? True (IgE-mediated) food allergy is much more likely in patients who have seasonal or perennial allergic rhinitis. Exceptions are (wasp/bee) venom and drug allergy, which occur similarly in atopic and non-atopic patients).

▷ Other questions should include family history (allergy is more common when there is an atopic parent), environmental history (exposure to furry animals, house dust mite) and occupation/hobbies.

Objective tests

There is controversy in the UK about the need for objective tests given that the treatment for the most commonly presenting problems (asthma and rhinitis) is rarely allergen specific and usually consists of a combination of bronchodilator and inhaled anti-inflammatory drugs (asthma) and anti-histamines and nasal anti-inflammatory drugs (rhinitis). However, patients often wish to develop some degree of non-pharmacological control of their symptoms and are keen to identify potential triggers and to institute avoidance measures where possible. Making a clear diagnosis is vital to avoid costly and time-consuming avoidance measures; for example, avoiding common foods in the absence of any measurable link between symptoms and exposure is stressful and associated with considerable morbidity. Similarly, avoiding penicillin to prevent anaphylaxis in a child with repeated chest infections because of an isolated childhood rash and no evidence of an IgE-mediated cause is costly and might have severe cost implications during hospital admissions in later life.

Skin prick tests and blood tests are available to identify an IgE-mediated mechanism in patients with allergic symptoms, or to exclude allergy in patients with atypical symptoms. They are both used to diagnose atopy, that is, the predisposition to develop allergic symptoms, and should not be interpreted as evidence of a causal relationship between exposure and symptoms unless the history is compatible with the test results.

Positive skin prick tests and blood tests demonstrate sensitisation to a particular allergen, although the magnitude of the response does not necessarily correlate with disease severity. As a rough guide, however, skin test responses greater than 6 mm in diameter and specific IgE levels of approximately 11 kUA/l (to seasonal and perennial allergens) are more likely to be associated with clinical symptoms on exposure to the relevant allergen.[9] There is a relatively good correlation between skin prick tests and blood tests for aero-allergens,[10] and so the choice of test is likely to be based on the nature of the symptoms, safety, availability of extracts, cost and operator expertise in the interpretation of results. Patients in whom there is a discrepancy between the clinical history and results of objective tests might benefit from referral to an allergist (see www.bsaci.org for details of allergy services).[11]

Skin prick tests

Skin prick testing is regarded as a routine diagnostic procedure in hospital allergy clinics but is under-used in general practice. In a recent survey of approximately 500 nurses who had completed a postgraduate course in allergy diagnosis and management only around 10 per cent went on to offer skin prick testing in general practice, despite being given full training in correct technique and interpretation.[12] Reasons included lack of GP support, inadequate funding and safety concerns. Safety still appears to be a major concern, although the procedure is well tolerated by patients and by nurses performing the tests.[13] Routine skin prick tests that are helpful to confirm or refute the presence of atopy (in the UK) are grass pollen, house dust mite (*Dermatophagoides pteronyssinus*), cat and dog, plus negative and positive controls. Anaphylaxis following skin prick tests to common aero-allergens has not been reported.[14] Skin prick tests for foods are less reliable than those for aero-allergens, resulting in a high rate of false positives.[15] Advantages of performing a skin prick test include the quick test time (15 mins), the speed and visibility of the reaction, which might be helpful in reinforcing avoidance advice, and the relatively low cost.

Specific IgE blood tests

Measurement of allergen-specific IgE antibodies present in the serum is an alternative and comparably reliable way of diagnosing atopy (specific IgE to common aero-allergens) when skin prick tests are not available.[16] They are particularly useful to test for allergens that carry the risk of adverse reactions if used as a skin prick test (e.g. food allergens, venom, penicillin), although all patients in whom IgE-mediated anaphylaxis is suspected should be referred for a specialist allergy opinion. Specific IgE testing can be arranged via the local biochemistry/pathology laboratory. An important point to remember when arranging a test is to ensure that a specific IgE test to a particular allergen(s) is requested; it is not helpful to request a total IgE as this is not a reliable indicator of atopic status. Requests should be accompanied by clinical information to allow the laboratory to offer appropriate advice on interpretation.

Rhinitis and allergic rhinitis

Rhinitis is a common problem in Western societies, affecting approximately 24 per cent of the UK adult population.[17] Rhinitis can be defined as a collection of symptoms including a runny and/or blocked nose, sneezing, itching (and sometimes postnasal drip or conjunctivitis) occurring for an hour or more on most days. Symptoms can be seasonal (hay fever), perennial, or perennial with seasonal exacerbations, and have been shown to differ in their allergic (atopic) state, clinical presentation and medical history. Seasonal symptoms are caused by allergy in approximately 80 per cent of cases, whereas perennial symptoms are allergic in nature only 50 per cent of the time.[17] Seasonal rhinitis is characterised by sneezing, itching and a high prevalence of diurnal variation in symptoms. Common triggers include dust, pollens and infections. By comparison, perennial rhinitis is characterised by a higher prevalence of nasal blockage and catarrh, and a lower prevalence of diurnal variation and pollen-related triggers. Subjects with seasonal rhinitis are more likely to be atopic (i.e. have positive skin prick tests or serum IgE tests to common aero-allergens) and to have eczema and a family history of hay fever than those without rhinitis. Those with perennial rhinitis are more likely to have past or current eczema or migraine, be wheezy or labelled asthmatic, or have a family history of nose trouble other than hay fever.[17] Other causes of rhinitis symptoms include infection (viral, bacterial), structural problems of the nose (e.g. deviation of the nasal septum and polyps) and, less commonly, endocrine problems (hypothyroidism) and iatrogenic disease (e.g. the combined oral contraceptive pill).

Impact of allergic rhinitis

Allergic rhinitis (including hay fever) is common and can have a big impact on daily activities. Research has shown that it might adversely affect concentration,[18] reduce productivity and impair exam performance[19] in adolescents. The high prevalence of hay fever among adolescents,[19] combined with that fact that GSCE and A-level exams take place at the peak of the grass pollen season, mean it is vital to consider strategies for managing hay fever symptoms in this age group proactively, and to encourage patients to take advantage of the broad range of treatments available.

What is the role of allergy?

Causes of rhinitis are varied, but for simplicity they can be broadly grouped under headings of allergy and non-allergy. Their symptoms are similar, but allergic rhinitis is characterised by sneezing and itching, whereas the commonest symptoms in non-allergic rhinitis are nasal blockage and postnasal drip. Although rhinitis is easy to treat using a structured approach, it is helpful to differentiate between allergic and non-allergic rhinitis as the treatments may differ. In practice, simple questions can help to identify the most likely cause and select the most appropriate treatment.

Accurate history-taking is of primary importance in establishing the role of allergy. However, a positive response to the question 'Do you get hay fever?' correlates to a positive allergy test (skin prick test or measurement of serum-specific IgE) approximately 75 per cent of the time.[20]

In general, rhinitis is more likely to be allergic in nature if a trigger can be identified, if symptoms include sneezing and itching, and if there are associated eye symptoms.

Treatment is, in the majority of sufferers, extremely effective. However, care needs to be taken to get the combination of treatments right and to ensure patients take them correctly and regularly.

Diagnosis of allergic rhinitis

When thinking about diagnosing allergic rhinitis, it is worth noting that the treatment is rarely allergen specific, the most effective treatment being a combination of antihistamine and topical anti-inflammatory drugs.[21] This means that there is limited value in identifying specific allergen triggers, and treatment should be based on treating specific symptoms such as nasal blockage or sneezing.

The probability of rhinitis symptoms being allergic in nature is significantly increased, however, if symptoms are triggered by animals or pollen, or if the patient has a personal history or a family history of allergy.[20] The need for a diagnostic test should therefore depend on whether or not the identification of an allergen trigger will influence the treatment decision.[22] Given the challenges in avoiding exposure to these allergen triggers, there is in most individuals little merit in identifying the underlying allergenic trigger. Empirical treatment is therefore justified as an initial step for rhinitis patients with a convincing history of allergy, that is, patients with a personal or family history of asthma, eczema or hay fever who have symptoms that occur within minutes of exposure and fit the pattern of histamine release in one or more target organs (i.e. redness, itching or swelling).

However, where avoidance is both effective and possible (in the case of food or drug allergy) or an allergen-specific treatment such as immunotherapy is being considered, then identification of the specific allergen trigger is essential, although, again, accurate history-taking is of primary importance in establishing the role of allergy and interpreting test results. The medical history, related to the nature and timing of the symptoms, trigger factors and evidence of personal and family history of allergic disease, should guide the need for, and choice of, diagnostic test.[23]

Management

Allergen avoidance

Airborne allergens such as grass pollen, house dust mite and cat allergen are virtually impossible to avoid effectively. There is little evidence to support allergen avoidance measures in adults[24,25] although complex interventions based on individual allergen sensitivities have shown some benefit in high-risk children.[26]

Pharmacological management of rhinitis

Guidelines recommend a combination of non-sedating antihistamines, long-acting topical nasal corticosteroids and anti-inflammatory eye drops.[21] Part of the management strategy should also be to arrange adequate follow-up and to encourage patient self-management for optimal symptom control.

▷ Patients with persistent nasal symptoms (particularly nasal blockage, itching and sneezing) should be treated with a nasal corticosteroid; once-daily preparations might aid compliance.

▷ Possible side effects include nose bleeds and nasal crusting, and are generally related to method of administration. Prescription of topical nasal sprays should always be accompanied by an explanation of device technique (see Figure 5.1); sniffing hard during administration should be avoided.

▷ Patients should be advised of the need for regular steroid treatment and advised that benefit might not be immediate. They should also be shown how to use nasal sprays (see Figure 5.1).

▷ Regular (daily) use is superior to PRN use, although PRN use is superior to placebo.

▷ Watery rhinorrhea tends to respond better to topical anti-cholinergic drugs rather than nasal corticosteroids.

▷ In patients whose symptoms remain uncontrolled, consider adding a non-sedating antihistamine.

▷ Antihistamines are less effective in the treatment of nasal blockage, although newer antihistamines such as desloratidine or fexofenadine might be helpful.

▷ Antihistamines are effective at reducing associated eye symptoms.

▷ In patients with seasonal symptoms, treatment should begin at least two weeks before symptoms are expected to start for maximal effect.

▷ Topical sodium cromoglycate should be added for uncontrolled eye symptoms (its use is contraindicated in contact lens wearers); topical H_1-antagonists should be considered in patients with isolated eye/nose symptoms. Corticosteroid eye drops should not be used unless supervised by an ophthalmologist because of the risks of side effects.

▷ Patients with rhinitis should be investigated for asthma and treated with bronchodilators and inhaled corticosteroids as appropriate.

▷ A follow-up visit allows identification of side effects that might affect compliance with treatment.

Figure 5.1 ○ *How to take aqueous nasal sprays*

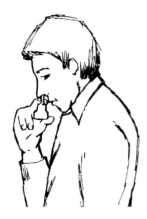

- Stand up, fixing the eyes on a point on the floor about 3 feet away.
- Using the right hand for the left nostril, and vice versa, insert the tip
- Use the required number of sprays according to instructions.
- Do not sniff! (Sniffing might result in the drug going to the stomach instead of the nose; this might be the biggest reason for treatment failure.)

Source: image copyright Education for Health, www.educationforhealth.org.uk.

The main reasons for treatment failure are likely to be poor compliance, poor nasal spray technique, or inadequate dosing. If symptoms persist despite optimal pharmacotherapy, or if the patient has exams or an important event coming up, a number of options are available.

Managing severe or uncontrolled symptoms

A short course of oral corticosteroids (e.g. 20 mg prednisolone daily for five days) is widely held to be effective for severe hay fever symptoms, although evidence is limited and unacceptable systemic side effects occur with prolonged use.

Although depot steroid injections are effective in controlling symptoms of severe hay fever,[11] there remains concern over their safety. Reported side effects include local effects such as post-injection flare, facial flushing and skin and fat atrophy; systemic complications are rare but include tissue atrophy.[27,28] Moreover, a persistent effect on bones or eyes cannot be excluded. Depot corticosteroid treatment for hay fever was found to cause avascular necrosis of both hips,[29] and fatalities related to intramuscular and intra-articular injections have been reported.[30]

Medico-legal issues related to the use of intramuscular corticosteroid treatment have arisen, and using these drugs to treat a condition for which alternative safe and effective treatments exist should be considered with caution.

Immunotherapy, or desensitisation, retains a role in the treatment of those with hay fever who are unresponsive to or cannot tolerate conventional pharmacotherapy. Subcutaneous immunotherapy has been shown to reduce symptoms by half and medication use by 80 per cent.[31] Long-term efficacy of immunotherapy following three years' treatment has also been demonstrated.[32]

Success depends on appropriate patient selection, that is, clinically mono-sensitive patients with identifiable IgE-mediated disease who do not respond to a combination of nasal steroids and antihistamines. Subcutaneous immunotherapy is only available from trained staff based in specialist centres. Sublingual immunotherapy is a safe and effective alternative[33] that can be prescribed in general practice, although, again, careful patient selection is required.

Anaphylaxis

Anaphylaxis is a relatively uncommon but potentially life-threatening condition. It can have significant long-term psychosocial implications for both individuals and their families.

Definition

Although the term was introduced over a hundred years ago now, there is still currently no universally accepted definition of anaphylaxis. A recent US-led initiative aiming to arrive at a consensus definition has however offered the following: 'Anaphylaxis is a severe, potentially fatal, systemic allergic reaction that occurs suddenly after contact with an allergy-causing substance.'[34]

Epidemiology

The lack of progress in arriving at a clinically and epidemiologically sound definition has hampered progress in developing an accurate understanding of the epidemiology of anaphylaxis; also contributing to this relative lack of progress has been the difficulties of mounting prospective studies investigating this acute, infrequent and short-lived attack. That said, some progress has been made and a recent international review of the literature by the Working Group of the American College of Allergy, Asthma and Immunology concluded that the overall frequency of episodes of anaphylaxis using current data lies between 30–60 cases per 100,000 person years at the lower end and 950 cases per 100,000 persons years at the higher end.[35] This report indicated a lifetime prevalence of between 50 and 2000 episodes/100,000 persons or 0.05–2.0 per cent. More recent UK primary care data concur with these estimates, indicating a lifetime age-standardised prevalence of a recorded diagnosis of anaphylaxis of 75.5 per 100,000 person years in 2005.[36] Calculations based on these data indicate that approximately 1 in 1333 of the English population or approximately 37,000 people have a medically recorded experience of anaphylaxis at some point in their lives. The limited data available on trends show that hospital admissions for anaphylaxis in England increased by 700 per cent during the period 1990–2004.[37, 38]

Triggers

Anaphylaxis can be triggered by any of a very broad range of factors, but factors that are most commonly identified include food, drugs and venom. The relative importance of these varies very considerably with age, with food being particularly important in children and medicinal products being much more common triggers in older people.[39] Virtually any food or class of drug can be implicated, although the classes of foods and drugs responsible for the majority of reactions are well described.[40] It is important to note that in many cases, despite extensive investigation, no known cause can be identified.

Diagnosis

The diagnosis is in the overwhelming majority of cases a clinical one, this being helped by knowledge of exposure to a known or suspected (allergic) trigger. Any of a number of symptoms may be present (see Table 5.2), the most common of which is cutaneous and/or mucosal involvement. The diagnosis of anaphylaxis is however crucially dependent on life-threatening features as manifested by respiratory and/or cardiovascular involvement.

Table 5.2 ○ *Clinical features of anaphylaxis*

Organ system affected	Symptoms and signs
Skin	Erythema, pruritis, urticaria and angioedema
Eyes	Injection of the conjunctiva, watery eyes and itching
Airways	Sneezing, rhinorrhoea, laryngeal oedema, cough, wheeze and dyspnoea
Gastrointestinal	Tongue swelling, abdominal cramps, vomiting and diarrhoea
Cardiovascular	Palpitations, light-headedness and collapse

Investigations

Measurement of mast cell tryptase might be useful in differentiating between anaphylaxis and other possible causes of an acute reaction. Tryptase levels rise rapidly shortly after anaphylaxis, peaking at about 1–2 hours post-mast cell degranulation, and then fall gradually over the next 4–6 hours.[41] The timing of the test is therefore important, but as this is of no value in the *acute* management of suspected cases of anaphylaxis, emergency treatment should not in any way be compromised.

Once fully recovered, all patients experiencing anaphylaxis should be investigated to identify trigger factors and, in the light of these investigations, be issued with advice on ways of minimising the risk of recurrence.

Management

Management can helpfully be considered in two stages: emergency management and longer-term care.

EMERGENCY MANAGEMENT

The Resuscitation Council UK recommends the ABCDE approach to the emergency management of all patients with suspected anaphylaxis. In essence, this focuses on assessment and if necessary treatment of the: **A**irway; **B**reathing; **C**irculation; **D**isability; and **E**xposure.[42] Key considerations in the emergency management of anaphylaxis are summarised in Figure 5.2. Particularly noteworthy is the need for early administration of IM adrenaline, which might be life saving.[43]

LONGER-TERM CARE

The longer-term needs of patients with anaphylaxis are all too often overlooked and this failure to appreciate the wider implications of living with a potentially life-threatening disorder can result in considerable psychosocial consequences and morbidity.[44] Creating individually tailored anaphylaxis management plans – which amongst other things provide written advice on known triggers and detailed recommendations on how to avoid these, and also what to do in an emergency situation – is one way of ensuring that at least some of the longer-term needs of people with anaphylaxis are met, although there is as yet limited research evidence to support this approach.[45] All patients at risk of recurrence of anaphylaxis should be issued with self-administered adrenaline and given detailed instructions on how

Figure 5.2 ○ *Anaphylaxis algorithm*

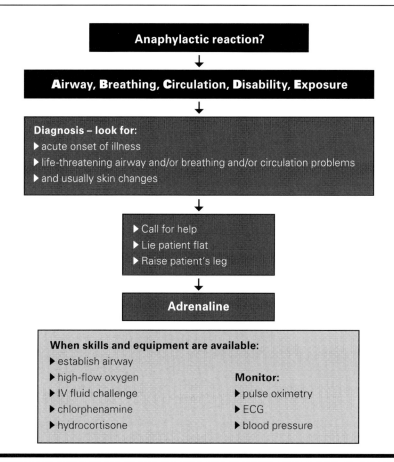

Anaphylactic reaction?

↓

Airway, Breathing, Circulation, Disability, Exposure

↓

Diagnosis – look for:
▶ acute onset of illness
▶ life-threatening airway and/or breathing and/or circulation problems
▶ and usually skin changes

↓

▶ Call for help
▶ Lie patient flat
▶ Raise patient's leg

↓

Adrenaline

When skills and equipment are available:
▶ establish airway
▶ high-flow oxygen   **Monitor:**
▶ IV fluid challenge   ▶ pulse oximetry
▶ chlorphenamine   ▶ ECG
▶ hydrocortisone   ▶ blood pressure

1. Life-threatening problems:

Airway ▶ swelling, hoarseness, stridor
Breathing ▶ rapid breathing, wheeze, fatigue, cyanosis, SpO2 <92%, confusion
Circulation ▶ pale, clammy, low blood pressure, faintness, drowsy/coma

2. Adrenaline (*give IM unless experienced with IV adrenaline*)
IM doses of 1:1000 adrenaline (repeat after 5 min if no better)

Adult ▶ 500 micrograms IM (0.5 ml)
Child more than 12 years ▶ 500 micrograms IM (0.5 ml)
Child 6–12 years ▶ 300 micrograms IM (0.3 ml)
Child less than 6 years ▶ 150 micrograms IM (0.15 ml)

Adrenaline IV to be given only by experienced specialists
Titrates: adults 50 micrograms; children 1 microgram/kg

3. IV fluid challenge:

Adult ▶ 500–1000 ml
Child ▶ crystalloid 20 ml/kg

Stop IV colloid
if this might be the cause
of anaphylaxis

	4. Chlorphenamine **(IM or slow IV)**	**5. Hydrocortisone** **(IM or slow IV)**
Adult or child more than 12 years ▶	10 mg	200 mg
Child 6–12 years ▶	5 mg	100 mg
Child 6 months to 6 years ▶	2.5 mg	50 mg
Child less than 6 months ▶ 250 micrograms/kg		25 mg

Source: copyright Resuscitation Council, www.resus.org.uk/pages/anaalgo.pdf.

89

and when to use this. Medic-alert jewellery that documents the condition and location of emergency treatment should also be considered.

Prognosis

The case fatality ratio of anaphylaxis is low, estimated at less than 1 per cent. Nonetheless, deaths do occur. Groups at particular risk are adolescents (possibly as a consequence of greater risk-taking behaviour) and those with a pre-existing history of asthma that is poorly controlled.[46,47]

Further self-assessment

A) Skin prick tests
Which of the following statements are correct?

1 ▷ Skin prick tests can be used to demonstrate sensitisation to an allergen.
2 ▷ Skin prick tests confirm a causal relationship with an allergen.
3 ▷ The magnitude of the skin response does not correlate with the severity of the allergic disease.
4 ▷ Skin prick testing is readily available in general practice.
5 ▷ Skin prick testing carries a high risk of severe anaphylaxis.

Key ▶ True – **1**, **3**.

B) Allergic rhinitis
Which of the following conditions are more common amongst patients with allergic rhinitis than in the normal population?

1 ▷ Asthma
2 ▷ Eczema
3 ▷ Family history of other nasal problems
4 ▷ Migraine
5 ▷ Nasal polyps

Key ▶ **1**, **2** and **3** are true.

References

1 • Kay A B. 100 years of 'allergy': can von Pirquet's word be rescued? *Clinical and Experimental Allergy* 2006; **36**: 555–9.

2 • Porter R. *The Greatest Benefit to Mankind* London: Harper Collins, 1997.

3 • Room A. *The Cassell Dictionary of Word Histories* London: Cassell, 1999.

4 • Peakman M, Vergani D. *Basic and Clinical Immunology* New York: Churchill, 1997.

5 • Kay A B. Principles and practice of diagnosis and treatment of allergic disease. In: A B Kay (ed.). *Allergy and Allergic Diseases* Oxford: Blackwell Science, 1997, pp. 1271–90.

6 • Jackson M. Allergy: the making of a modern plague *Clinical and Experimental Allergy* 2001; **31**: 1665–71.

7 • Gell P G H, Coombs R R A. The classification of allergic reactions underlying disease. In: P G H Gell, R R A Coombs (eds). *Clinical Aspects of Immunology* Oxford: Blackwell Scientific Productions, 1963, pp. 317–37.

8 • Gruchalla R S, Pirmohamed M. Antibiotic allergy *New England Journal of Medicine* 2006; **354(6)**: 601–9.

9 • Pastorello E A, Incorvaia C, Ortolani C, *et al*. Studies on the relationship between the level of specific IgE antibodies and the clinical expression of allergy: I. Definition of levels distinguishing patients with symptomatic from patients with asymptomatic allergy to common aeroallergens *Journal of Allergy and Clinical Immunology* 1995; **96**: 580–7.

10 • Williams P B, Dolen W K, Koepke J W, *et al*. Comparison of skin testing and three in vitro assays for specific IgE in the clinical evaluation of immediate hypersensitivity *Annals of Allergy* 1992; **68**: 35–45.

11 • Royal College of Physicians and Royal College of Pathologists. Good allergy practice: standards of care for providers and purchasers of allergy services within the National Health Service *Clinical and Experimental Allergy* 1995; **25**: 586–95.

12 • Walker S M. Evaluating allergy practice *NRTC Bulletin* 2001; 8.

13 • Sibbald B, Barnes G, Durham S R. Skin prick testing in general practice: a pilot study *Journal of Advanced Nursing* 1997; **26**: 537–42.

14 • Reid M J, Lockey R F, Turkeltaub P C, *et al*. Survey of fatalities from skin testing and immunotherapy 1985–1989 *Journal of Allergy and Clinical Immunology* 1993; **92**: 6–15.

15 • Sampson H A, Albergo R. Comparison of the results of skin tests, R AST, and double-blind placebo-controlled food challenges in children with atopic dermatitis *Journal of Allergy and Clinical Immunology* 1984; **74**: 26–33.

16 • Witteman A M, Stapel P O, Perdok G J, *et al*. The relationship between R AST and skin test results in patients with asthma or rhinitis: a quantitative study with purified major allergens *Journal of Allergy and Clinical Immunology* 1996; **97**: 16–25.

17 • Sibbald B, Rink E. Epidemiology of seasonal and perennial rhinitis: clinical presentation and clinical history *Thorax* 1991; **46**: 895–901.

18 • Juniper E F, Guyatt G H. Development and testing of a new measure of health status for clinical trials in rhinoconjunctivitis *Clinical and Experimental Allergy* 1990; **21**: 77–83.

19 • Walker S, Khan-Wasti S, Fletcher M, *et al*. Seasonal allergic rhinitis is associated with a detrimental impact on exam performance in UK teenagers: case-control study *Journal of Allergy and Clinical Immunology* 2007; **120(2)**: 381–7.

20 • Kilpeläinen M, Terho E O, Helenius H, *et al*. Validation of a new questionnaire on asthma, allergic rhinitis, and conjunctivitis in young adults *Allergy* 2001; **56**: 377–84.

21 • Price D, Bond C, Bouchard J, *et al*. International Primary Care Respiratory Group (IPCRG) Guidelines: management of allergic rhinitis *Primary Care Respiratory Journal* 2006; **15**: 58–70.

22 • Walker S M, Morton C, Sheikh A. Diagnosing allergy in primary care: are the history and clinical examination sufficient? *Primary Care Respiratory Journal* 2006; **15**: 219–21.

23 • Gendo K, Larson E B. Evidence-based diagnostic strategies for evaluating suspected allergic rhinitis *Annals of Internal Medicine* 2004; **140(4)**: 278–89.

24 • Sheikh A, Hurwitz B. House dust mite avoidance measures for perennial allergic rhinitis: a systematic review of efficacy *British Journal of General Practice* 2003; **53(489)**: 318–22.

25 • Gøtszche PC, Johansen H K, Schmidt L M, *et al*. House dust mite control measures for asthma *Cochrane Database of Systematic Reviews* CD001187. 2004.

26 • Morgan W J, Crain E F, Gruchalla R S, *et al*. Inner-City Asthma Study Group. Results of a home-based environmental intervention among urban children with asthma *New England Journal of Medicine* 2004; **351(11)**: 1068–80.

27 • Dyment P G. Local atrophy following triamcinalone injection *Pediatrics* 1970; **46(1)**: 136–7.

28 • Jacobs M B. Local subcutaneous atrophy after corticosteroid injection *Postgraduate Medical Journal* 1986; **80(4)**: 159–60.

29 • Nasser S, Ewan P. Lesson of the week: depot corticosteroid treatment for hayfever causing avascular necrosis of both hips *British Medical Journal* 2001; **322**: 1589–91.

30 • Ewan P W. Anaphylaxis *British Medical Journal* 1998 9; **316(7142)**: 1442–5.

31 • Walker S M, Pajno G, Torres Lima M, *et al*. Grass pollen immunotherapy for seasonal rhinitis and asthma: a randomised controlled trial *Journal of Allergy and Clinical Immunology* 2001; **107**: 87–93.

32 • Durham S R, Walker S M, Varga E-M, *et al*. Long-term clinical efficacy of grass pollen immunotherapy *New England Journal of Medicine* 1999; **341**: 468–75.

33 • Dahl R, Kapp A, Colombo G, *et al*. Efficacy and safety of sublingual immunotherapy with grass allergen tablets for seasonal allergic rhinoconjunctivitis *Journal of Allergy and Clinical Immunology* 2006; **118(2)**: 434–40.

34 • Sampson H A, Muñoz-Furlong A, Campbell R, *et al*. Second Symposium on the Definition and Management of Anaphylaxis: summary report – Second National Institute of Allergy and Infectious Disease/Food Allergy and Anaphylaxis Network Symposium *Annals of Emergency Medicine* 2006; **47(4)**: 373–80.

35 • Lieberman P, Camargo C, Bohlke K, *et al*. Epidemiology of anaphylaxis: findings of the American College of Allergy, Asthma and Immunology Epidemiology of Anaphylaxis Working Group *Annals of Allergy, Asthma and Immunology* 2006; **97**: 596–602.

36 • Sheikh A, Hippisley-Cox J, Newton J, *et al*. Trends in national incidence, lifetime prevalence and adrenaline prescribing for anaphylaxis in England *Journal of the Royal Society of Medicine* 2008; **101**: 139–43.

37 • Gupta R, Sheikh A, Strachan D, *et al*. Increasing hospital admissions for systemic allergic disorders in England: analysis of national admissions data *British Medical Journal* 2003; **327**: 1142–3.

38 • Gupta R, Sheikh A, Strachan D P, *et al*. Time trends in allergic disorders in the UK *Thorax* 2006; **62(1)**: 91–6.

39 • Alves B, Sheikh A. Age-specific aetiology of anaphylaxis: a study of routine hospital admission data in England *Archives of Disease in Childhood* 2001; **85(4)**: 349.

40 • Ewan P, 1998.

41 • Schwartz L B. Diagnostic value of tryptase in anaphylaxis and mastocytosis *Immunology and Allergy Clinics of North America* 2006; **26**: 451–63.

42 • Soar J, Pumphrey R, Cant A, *et al.*; Working Group of the Resuscitation Council (UK). Emergency treatment of anaphylactic reactions: statement paper guidelines for healthcare providers *Resuscitation* 2008; **77(2)**: 157–69.

43 • Sheikh A, Shehata Y A, Brown S G, *et al.* Adrenaline for the treatment of anaphylaxis: Cochrane systematic review *Allergy* 2009; **64(2)**: 204–12.

44 • Akeson N, Worth A, Sheikh A. The psychosocial impact of anaphylaxis on young people and their parents *Clinical and Experimental Allergy* 2007; **37**: 1213–20.

45 • Choo K, Sheikh A. Action plans for the long-term management of anaphylaxis: systematic review of effectiveness *Clinical and Experimental Allergy* 2007; **37**: 1090–4.

46 • Pumphrey R S. Lessons for management of anaphylaxis from a study of fatal reactions *Clinical and Experimental Allergy* 2000; **30**: 1144–50.

47 • Pumphrey R S H, Gowland M H. Further fatal allergic reactions to food in the United Kingdom, 1999–2006 *Journal of Allergy and Clinical Immunology* 2007; **119**: 1018–19.

93

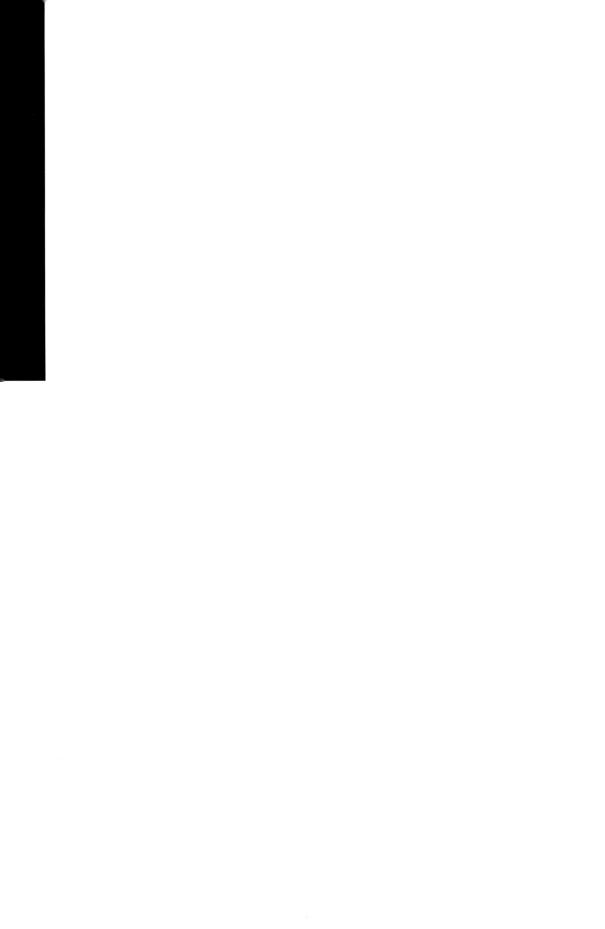

Respiratory diseases of childhood

6

Iain Small

Chapter aims

This chapter explores the common causes of respiratory problems in child-hood, considering their diagnosis and management.

Learning outcomes

▷ To understand how general practitioners (GPs) establish a diagnosis in children with respiratory symptoms.
▷ To explore some common diseases of children as they present in primary care.
▷ To consider the role of the GP in treating and supporting children with respiratory disease and their families.

Initial self-assessment

A) Which of the following statements is true about children with bronchiolitis?

1 ▷ Bronchiolitis typically presents in children aged 4 to 6.
2 ▷ Respiratory syncytial virus (RSV) accounts for about 50 per cent of cases of bronchiloitis.
3 ▷ RSV-positive bronchiolitis has been linked to subsequent asthma.
4 ▷ All children with bronchiolitis should be admitted to hospital for investigation.

Key ▶ **3**

B) Raj, a 10-month-old boy with fever, tachypnoea and wheezing, is presented to you at the out-of-hours GP service. Consider:

1 ▷ What factors in the history would you question and what would you look for on examination?

2 ▷ What conditions would you consider in your differential diagnosis?

Introduction

It's a child's job to cause problems for his or her parents. Anyone who has gone through the experience of parenthood will recognise the understatement. In addition, anyone who has spent time looking after children, examining, investigating and treating them, will recognise that they are not simply mini-adults. Children present with their own unique medical problems, with illnesses sometimes only found in their age group, or they might present with a range of symptoms completely at odds with the effects of the same pathology in adults. It is also true, of course, that many long-term or lifelong conditions might first become manifest, if not at birth, then in the growing child. This is certainly true in the respiratory field.

Amongst the range of causes for respiratory illness in children, we find:

▷ congenital
▷ genetic
▷ pre-term birth-related
▷ infection
▷ allergy
▷ neoplasm
▷ trauma.

If you add to this the concern of the clinician to intervene early, to try to limit the effects of pathology on developing respiratory structures, and his or her wish to avoid the impact of the side effects of therapies, in a kind of balancing act of many evils, then we are presented with a challenge that would vex most paediatric specialists. This, however, is the everyday work of the new generalist, be they practice nurse or GP in primary care in the twenty-first century.

In this chapter we will concentrate on the common causes of respiratory illness in children, dealing with asthma, its differential diagnosis, and its relationship to common infectious illnesses such as RSV. We will also consider other significant potential diagnoses in children presenting with cough and wheeze, such as cystic fibrosis (CF) and bacterial sepsis, and look at methods that can be used to tease out the true diagnosis, particularly in pre-school children.

Of course, when faced with such challenges, the wise clinician will revert to those techniques he or she learned whilst training. Although modern primary care has a range of consultation models for every occasion, perhaps in the case of the breathless or wheezy child the following time-honoured skills are worth remembering:

▷ history-taking
▷ examination
▷ investigation
▷ establishing a diagnosis
▷ treatment trials
▷ clinical review.

Establishing a diagnosis in children with respiratory symptoms

History-taking

It is, of course, stating the obvious to point out that small children are unable to give a history of their presenting complaint. The value of the consultation to both patient and clinician should not be underestimated, both in terms of giving useful clinical information, and helping to establish and cement the relationship between the parties, at a time in a family's life where anxiety is often all too easily generated. Establishing rapport at this stage can impact on future concordance, as can the patient or parent's understanding of the disease, their belief system, and their feeling of being actively involved in management.

Other problems in taking a history from this group of the population are self-evident; the frequency of reported symptoms, and their severity, is observer dependent, with a potential for over- and under-estimation. This might be inadvertent – parents failing to report accurately the child's night-time symptoms, for example – or might be part of a wider and more complex psychological or social problem within the family unit. In these circumstances, the frequency of a child's symptoms might be influenced by many factors, including parental anxiety, socioeconomic circumstances, family size (including number of parents), ethnicity and cultural norms.

Important factors to consider when taking a history in children are:

▶ presenting complaint
  ▷ cough

- ▷ wheeze
- ▷ breathlessness
- ▷ cyanosis
- ▶ associated symptoms
  - ▷ diurnal variation
  - ▷ sputum production
  - ▷ atopy
  - ▷ failure to thrive
- ▶ family history
  - ▷ genetic
  - ▷ atopy
  - ▷ position of child in family and siblings
  - ▷ ethnicity and travel
- ▶ birth history
  - ▷ pre-term
  - ▷ trauma
  - ▷ early feeding difficulties
- ▶ medication
  - ▷ over the counter (OTC)
  - ▷ allergies
  - ▷ response to treatments already given
  - ▷ immunisation history.

Examination

The clinical examination of the screaming child is never easy. Gaining the confidence of a miserable 18-month-old, held in the arms of an anxious parent, in the hostile environment of the consultation room is a challenging task, and even the most experienced clinician will find it difficult to identify the exact source of abnormal breath sounds. The few extra minutes needed to befriend a child when it accompanies a parent or guardian for other reasons might prove invaluable in establishing rapport in advance of the child's own illness presentation. Important factors to consider when examining children are:

- ▶ failure to thrive
  - ▷ plot the child's height and weight
  - ▷ evidence of poor nutritional status
  - ▷ evidence of recent change

▶ abnormal thoracic shape
  ▷ pectus excavatum
  ▷ Harrison's sulcus
▶ ear, nose and throat (ENT) examination
  ▷ lymphadenopathy
  ▷ tonsils and adenoids
  ▷ secretory otitis media
▶ auscultation
  ▷ presence of audible wheeze
  ▷ localised signs
  ▷ transmitted noise
▶ developmental assessment.

Establishing a working diagnosis

Asthma can present in very small children. It is important to remember, however, that not all that coughs or wheezes is asthma, and that establishing such a diagnosis requires careful consideration of the signs and symptoms demonstrated by the patient.

Work performed in primary care suggests that less than 20 per cent of children in this age group, given an asthma diagnosis, are indeed suffering from true allergic asthma, in which symptoms persist beyond the age of 10 years. The most common differential diagnosis is RSV bronchiolitis, which can cause a similar clinical pattern of symptoms to asthma, particularly in the under-2s. Chronic bacterial sepsis must also be considered as a differential, as must specific infections such as pertussis, and, of course, CF.

Common diseases of children presenting in primary care

Asthma

Although many small children will present with asthma-like symptoms, recent long-term follow-up studies would suggest that the following factors have a predictive value in making the diagnosis:

▷ atopy
▷ parental history of atopy (especially asthma)
▷ the presence of persisting respiratory symptoms.

Children with asthma are unlikely to have persisting wet cough, digestive symptoms or significant failure to thrive. Hearing wheeze on auscultation is always significant, and its absence (in the symptomatic child) should always be noted and considered. When this happens, other potential causes are more likely, and a return to the history might be valuable.

Measuring obstruction is very difficult in this age group. Recent improvements in computer-assisted spirometry might hold some promise. Where spirometry has been tried, interestingly, the $FEV_{0.5}$ might be more accurate than FEV_1.

Although none of these techniques is likely to gain widespread use in clinical practice in primary care, the importance of establishing a good working diagnosis of asthma cannot be over-emphasised. Peak flow measurement is inaccurate when used in children under the age of 5 years. The primary care clinician is often left considering a combination of good history, the absence of pointers towards other disease, and a trial of treatment, a strategy supported by national and international guidelines, but which calls for regular and effective review, especially in the face of persisting or resistant symptoms. In all cases, a full consideration of differential diagnosis should be remembered.

Respiratory syncytial virus

RSV infection accounts for 70 per cent or more of all cases of infantile bronchiolitis,[1] and is often associated with recurring episodes of wheeze. There is mounting evidence to suggest that infection in early life increases the risk of developing a kind of reactive airway disease (RAD) later in childhood. Children admitted to hospital with RSV bronchiolitis in infancy face a significantly increased risk of recurrent wheezing and allergy, which might persist beyond school entry, until at least the age of 7 years. This risk is independent of hereditary factors. To add confusion, RSV bronchiolitis has also been linked to subsequent asthma, either directly (as a cause for asthma), or through a shared common predisposition.

Our current understanding is that both genetic and environmental factors determine the type of immune response a child will mount towards RSV infection and that this response, in turn, might affect the development of the control mechanisms involved in the regulation of airway tone, and thus subsequent bronchospasm. How this relationship is relevant to the individual child, with reference to its RSV exposure and emerging asthma, might depend on individual phenotypes, with one group developing an asthma pattern, the other post-bronchiolitic wheeze (or RAD).

TREATMENT OPTIONS

ASTHMA AND PERI-VIRAL WHEEZE

Inhaled bronchodilators are the treatment of choice for small children suf-fering from episodic and persistent wheeziness, whether caused by simple viral infection or RSV. Both beta-agonists and anti-cholinergic drugs can be used, preferably through a large volume spacer. Since lung deposition is poor in this age group, the number of pressurised metered dose inhaler (pMDI) puffs given per dose must reflect this. The role of corticosteroids is more contentious. In the USA, oral prednisolone has been used, although there is mixed evidence as to its effectiveness. Its use (and that of parenteral steroid) is not supported by evidence-based guidelines such as SIGN (Scottish Inter-collegiate Guidelines Network).[2] Parent-initiated prednisolone therapy in these children might even increase the risk of hospital admission.

Inhaled corticosteroids have a well-established record in the treatment of asthma, but there is little evidence for their use in very small children. The primary care clinician faces a dilemma between the potential benefits and risks of treatment. Benefits might include short-term symptom control and longer-term disease modification as measured by FEV_1, whilst the potential risks of exposing the developing lung to this group of drugs is unknown. An agreed trial of treatment for a period of 4–6 weeks, at low dose, with acknowledged anticipated outcomes might be considered, particularly where there are recognised predictive factors for asthma.

Work in older children using what most clinicians would view as accepta-ble doses (<400 mcg budesonide equivalent) demonstrates a reassuring safety profile, particularly in terms of final height, growth velocity and weight.

The role of leukotriene receptor antagonists (LTRAs) is likewise poorly defined in younger children. There is undoubtedly a group of patients who respond well to these drugs, for whom they will be steroid sparing, but their role as a monotherapy is not supported by the breadth of available evidence. They may be considered as the first-choice anti-inflammatory in children with asthma, where the use of inhaled corticosteroids is considered inadvis-able, and provision for this option exists within guidelines.

EFFECTIVE DRUG DELIVERY

It remains tempting to many clinicians to go for the oral route when con-templating treatment options in small children. This can result in exposure to high doses of drugs such as short-acting beta-agonists (SABAs). Even infants can be treated with pMDIs using a spacer. Both SABAs and inhaled corticosteroids should be given this way.

In children with acute asthma, there is an increasing trend towards the use of multi-dosing with beta-agonists through spacers.[3] In the absence of life-threatening features of asthma, multi-dosing should be recommended to parents and carers of children with asthma. Asthma UK's 'First aid asthma plan for children and young people in your care' is a useful tool in this regard.

Where a child is suffering from life-threatening asthma, nebulisers should, when used, be driven through high-flow oxygen, as opposed to compressed air.

Bacterial sepsis

The trend towards the accurate diagnosis of asthma in children has led, over a generation, to the virtual disappearance of terms such as 'wheezy bronchitis' and 'chest infection'. As is often the case, however, medicine tends to come full circle. Today, there is increasing evidence that some pre-school children with chronic productive (or wet) cough might indeed have persisting bacterial sepsis in their airways. Good history-taking, together with clinical examination, should help to identify such children.

TREATMENT OPTIONS

In the absence of factors pointing to a diagnosis of asthma, CF, or other significant disease, prolonged courses of antibiotics (such as macrolides) can be very successful in achieving complete cure of such patients. Antibiotic treatment may need to be given for periods up to 3 months, and due consideration to the diagnosis (including specialist referral) should be given.

Cystic fibrosis

CF is the most common life-threatening, recessively inherited disease of Caucasian populations.[4] The carrier rate is 1 in 25 and the incidence is 1 in 2500 live births. In the UK and North America, there are reports of CF in children of Asian origin, but it is rare in those of Afro-Caribbean origin. At the date of publication, up-to-date, accurate figures are difficult to give, but data from 1992 suggested that there were over 6500 people with CF in the UK with 65 per cent under 16 years (much of the data given here comes from *Standards for the Clinical Care of Children and Adults with Cystic Fibrosis in the UK 2001*, a Cystic Fibrosis Trust publication[5]).

Given that there are just over 300 births of affected children per year, and approximately 160 deaths, this figure will have risen substantially. The author leaves the reader to do his or her own arithmetic.

Although many patients with CF survive into adult life, it remains the case that children and adolescents die as a consequence of the respiratory and metabolic consequences of this multi-system disease.

The genetic mutation in CF affects the cell membrane's chloride channel, resulting in faulty regulation of salt and water movement across the membrane, with a consequent thickening of secretions, particularly in the respiratory and digestive tracts. In the lung this results in impaired clearance of micro-organisms, leading to bronchial damage, bronchiectasis and eventually death from respiratory failure.

PRESENTATION

The majority of patients present in early childhood with respiratory tract infections that are slow to clear. Persistent intestinal malabsorption and failure to thrive are also common presentations. About 15 per cent of children with CF present at birth with meconium ileus.

Unfortunately, in the UK, up to 10 per cent of patients have their diagnosis delayed until adult life, a situation that should change with the introduction of routine screening, by way of the postnatal Guthrie Test, which has been available in Scotland, Northern Ireland and Wales for many years.

Most of the morbidity and more than 90 per cent of the mortality in CF is due to chronic pulmonary sepsis and its complications. The newborn infant with CF has normal lungs, with only minor obstructive changes to the submucosal glands of the trachea and major bronchi. Bacterial infection (*Staphylococcus aureus* and *Haemophilus influenzae*) occurs early, possibly with non-infective inflammatory changes preceding colonisation. Eventually, chronic infection, particularly with *Pseudomonas aeruginosa*, is a significant complication, and the greatest challenge to both doctor and patient.

THE ROLE OF PRIMARY CARE IN CF

The role of the primary care clinician is to consider the diagnosis, to refer early (for formal diagnosis by sweat testing), to support the family, and to act as a signpost towards other sources of information and support for patient and family. In addition, the GP is likely to become involved in genetic counselling. Making a diagnosis is not always easy, and the cardinal rule of considering the diagnosis of CF when patients fail to respond to conventional treatment is wise, especially in the presence of failure to thrive.

Early diagnosis and treatment might have a profound influence on a child's long-term prognosis, and, as a result, existing siblings should be sweat tested, as should subsequent siblings when newborn (bearing in mind that testing in the newborn might prove inconclusive).

CF is a multi-system disease requiring a holistic approach to care. Care should aim to prevent, for as long as possible, chronic infection and later stabilise the pulmonary infections to minimise deterioration in respiratory function and to maintain a good nutritional state.

It is now generally agreed that a team of trained, experienced health professionals in a specialist CF centre best provides this type of care, with the GP assuming a supportive role.

Other common respiratory conditions in primary care

Other important differential diagnoses that need to be considered in the child with respiratory symptoms, in this age group, are pertussis infection and, increasingly, tuberculosis (TB). Multi-drug-resistant and extreme drug-resistant TB are rare conditions, but can have a devastating impact on a child, family, and indeed the public health of an area.

With an increasingly mobile population, and increasing media scrutiny of immunisations and their safety, the wise clinician will pay particular attention to these factors when taking a history, especially when presented with a child with persisting cough. He or she should seek to exclude whooping cough and TB as a potential diagnosis in those at risk. In primary care the wise clinician will consider these, especially when faced with a child in whom the usual evidence for asthma is lacking. Specific factors such as ethnicity and previous travel, weight loss, socioeconomic status and special risk exposure are worth considering, and the extended primary care team (including social services and education) might provide valuable information.

In addition, respiratory symptoms might be due to inhaled foreign body, congenital abnormalities, such as tracheo-oesophageal fistula, immuno-deficiency state (either idiopathic or acquired) and, rarely, neoplasm, particularly in the mediastinum.

All children with persisting difficult symptoms should be referred for specialist advice where diagnostic and therapeutic doubts arise.

Summary

Children often present with a collection of problems, which include cough, wheeze, poor feeding, and sometimes choking and vomiting. Primary care clinicians in the UK are faced with the difficult, and at times impossible, challenge of working out the cause of this common symptom set.

Furthermore, having postulated a potential diagnosis, they face the unenviable task of deciding between a group of treatments that might be unproven, unlicensed, partially effective, and difficult to deliver.

Finally, this treatment needs to be given to a child whose therapeutic response might be unpredictable, unmeasurable, and occasionally unnoticed. We do all of this, whilst carrying with us the fears and anxiety of parents, colleagues and self, with inconclusive guidelines based on a scarcity of evidence, in a consultation that might last 5–10 minutes, and might take place in a badly lit, smoke-filled tenement flat, in the almost inevitable company of an angry dog.

Further self-assessment

Cystic fibrosis

Which of the following statements are true of CF?

1 ▷ CF is the commonest recessively inherited disease.
2 ▷ CF is common in all racial groups.
3 ▷ CF can be detected using a neonatal screening test.
4 ▷ CF is a condition that should always be treated in secondary care.

Key ▶ **1, 3**.

Resources

Reece A, Davies F. *Spotting the Sick Child* (DVD) University Hospital of Leicester and Royal College of Paediatrics and Child Health, 2004.

References

1 • Anderson LJ, Heilman CA. Protective and disease-enhancing immune responses to respiratory syncytial virus *Journal of Infectious Diseases* 1995; **171**: 1–7.

2 • British Thoracic Society and Scottish Intercollegiate Guidelines Network. *British Guideline on the Management of Asthma* (SIGN Guideline 101) Edinburgh: SIGN, 2008.

3 • National Institute for Health and Clinical Excellence. *Guidance on the Use of Inhaler Systems (Devices) in Children under the Age of 5 Years with Chronic Asthma* (Technology Appraisal 10) London: NICE, 2000.

4 • Vallance H, Ford J. Carrier testing for autosomal-recessive disorders *Critical Reviews in Clinical Laboratory Sciences* 2003; **20**: 473–97.

5 • The CF Trust's Clinical Standards and Accreditation Group. *Standards for the Clinical Care of Children and Adults with Cystic Fibrosis in the UK 2001* Bromley: CFT, 2001.

Breathlessness and cough

7

Yvonne Henderson and Rachel Booker

Chapter aims

This chapter aims to enable you to understand the complex symptom of breathlessness. It discusses the key components of a respiratory assessment and their role in helping to reach a diagnosis. It examines the causes of acute and chronic breathlessness and cough, and highlights the impact of breathlessness in end-stage disease.

Learning outcomes

At the end of this chapter you will be able to:

▷ understand the different components of a respiratory assessment and their role in assisting in diagnosing the cause of breathlessness
▷ understand the respiratory, cardiac and other causes of acute breathlessness
▷ understand the respiratory, cardiac and other causes of chronic breathlessness
▷ recognise dysfunctional breathing
▷ understand the causes and management of acute and chronic cough
▷ recognise the impact of breathlessness in end-stage disease.

Initial self-assessment

Which of the following clinical findings would suggest life-threatening asthma?

  A ▷ Bradycardia
  B ▷ Confusion
  C ▷ Cyanosis
  D ▷ Respiratory rate of 24 breaths per minute
  E ▷ Tachycardia

Key ▶ **A**, **B**, **C**.

Which of the following conditions are significant risk factors for acute left ventricular failure?

A ▷ Asthma

B ▷ Congenital heart disease

C ▷ Coronary heart disease

D ▷ Hypertension

E ▷ Hyperlipidaemia

Key ▶ **B, C, D**.

Which of the following drugs are recognised as causing drug-induced interstitial lung disease?

A ▷ Amiodarone

B ▷ Amlodipine

C ▷ Methotrexate

D ▷ Nitrofurantoin

E ▷ Trimethoprim

Key ▶ **A, C, D**.

Introducing breathlessness

Breathlessness is a very common but complex subjective symptom. It has many different causes and is indicative of a wide variety of conditions.

Becoming breathless on exertion is a normal physiological response to increased activity. In some people, however, breathlessness is an abnormal event, arising more frequently or more severely than would be expected. Abnormal breathlessness can be an important indication of:

▷ cardiac disease or dysfunction (e.g. left ventricular failure, valvular heart disease) and circulatory disorders (e.g. pulmonary embolism)

▷ respiratory disease or dysfunction (e.g. pneumothorax, asthma)

▷ neurological disease causing weakness of respiratory muscles (e.g. lower motor neurone disease, myasthenia gravis, Guillain-Barré syndrome)

▷ systemic disorder (e.g. hyperthyroidism, diabetic ketoacidosis, anaemia)

▷ psychological factors (e.g. panic attacks)

▷ dysfunctional breathing patterns (e.g. chronic hyperventilation syndrome)

▷ lifestyle factors (e.g. obesity hypoventilation syndrome).

Many different terms are used to describe the physical sensation of breathlessness, shown in Table 7.1 below:

Table 7.1 ○ *Terms relating to the physical sensation of breathlessness*

Dyspnoea	Awareness of increased respiratory effort that is perceived as unpleasant or inappropriate
Tachypnoea	Increased breathing rate
Hyperpnoea	Increased rate and depth of breathing
Orthopnoea	Breathlessness when lying down
Paroxysmal nocturnal dyspnoea	Being woken at night by breathlessness

Breathlessness is a very subjective symptom but it is important to quantify the degree of breathlessness as this is one of the most frequently used indicators of response to treatment.

The Medical Research Council (MRC) dyspnoea scale allows patients to rate their breathlessness according to the activity that induces it. The scale is shown below:

1 ▷ not troubled by breathlessness except on strenuous exercise
2 ▷ short of breath when hurrying or walking up a slight hill
3 ▷ walks slower than contemporaries on the level because of breathlessness, or has to stop for breath when walking at own pace
4 ▷ stops for breath after walking for 100 m or after a few minutes on the level
5 ▷ too breathless to leave the house, or breathless when dressing or undressing. Breathless at rest.

Alternatively a simple visual analogue scale might be appropriate. The MRC scale has the advantage that it can be coded onto practice clinical computer systems and be easily communicated to colleagues when referring patients.

Key points

▶ Observation of the patient begins as he or she enters the room.
▶ A systematic approach should be adopted that looks at the face, hands, pulse, lower limbs and ankles, skin, chest shape and movement.

▶ Auscultation of the lungs should identify breath sounds and additional sounds. Additional sounds include crackle, wheezes, rhonchi and pleural rub, all of which aid in diagnosis.

▶ Auscultation of the heart can be used to detect murmurs and additional heart sounds that are indicative of pathology.

▶ The severity of breathlessness can be assessed using the MRC dyspnoea scale or a simple visual analogue scale.

Causes of acute breathlessness

Respiratory causes of acute breathlessness

ASTHMA

Asthma causes airflow obstruction. It is characterised by airway inflammation and smooth-muscle dysfunction, resulting in bronchial hyper-responsiveness and constriction. Asthma is variable and the airflow obstruction is reversible, spontaneously or with treatment.[1]

Exercise is a common trigger and breathlessness on exertion is a key feature of uncontrolled asthma. During an acute exacerbation minimal exertion can produce disabling breathlessness.

The clinical features of acute exacerbations of asthma in adults are shown in Table 7.2.

Table 7.2 ○ *Clinical features of acute asthma*

Moderate asthma exacerbation	Increasing asthma symptoms PEF > 50–75% best or predicted No features of acute severe asthma
Acute severe asthma	PEF 33–50% predicted Inability to complete a sentence in one breath Respiratory rate > 25 breaths/min Heart rate > 110 beats/min
Life-threatening asthma	PEF < 33% best or predicted Silent chest Cyanosis Feeble respiratory effort Bradycardia Dysrhythmia Hypotension Exhaustion Confusion Collapse

Source: adapted from BTS and SIGN.[1]

The priorities for the emergency management of an acute attack of asthma are:

▷ bronchodilators
▷ oxygen to correct hypoxaemia
▷ oral corticosteroids.[1]

ACUTE EXACERBATION OF CHRONIC OBSTRUCTIVE PULMONARY DISEASE (AECOPD)

The natural history of chronic obstructive pulmonary disease (COPD) is punctuated by increasingly severe and frequent exacerbations. These can present with a variety of symptoms and are defined as:

a sustained worsening of the patient's symptoms from his or her usual stable state that is beyond normal day-to-day variations, and is acute in onset. Commonly reported symptoms are worsening breathlessness, cough, increased sputum production and change in sputum colour. The change in these symptoms often necessitates a change in medication.[2]

Many patients with COPD also have co-morbid conditions, particularly cardiovascular disease, and there are other conditions that present with similar symptoms. These include:

▷ pneumonia
▷ pneumothorax
▷ pulmonary embolism
▷ left ventricular failure and pulmonary oedema
▷ pleural effusion
▷ lung cancer.

A severe AECOPD will have one or more of the following features:

▷ severe dyspnoea (limiting activity)
▷ tachypnoea
▷ pursed-lip breathing
▷ accessory muscle use
▷ acute confusion
▷ new-onset cyanosis
▷ new onset or acute worsening of peripheral oedema
▷ marked reduction in activities of daily living.

The diagnosis is made on the basis of the clinical presentation. If there are features of a severe exacerbation pulse oximetry is useful, but, unlike asthma, the peak expiratory flow rate rarely adds any relevant information to the clinical assessment.

Respiratory failure is a potential complication of AECOPD in patients with moderate and severe COPD.

Red flags: features of respiratory failure

▶ Central cyanosis (bluish tongue and mucous membranes).

▶ Tachycardia – dysrhythmias are also common when hypoxaemia is severe.

▶ Tachypnoea.

▶ Hypertension.

▶ Altered mental state – confusion, agitation or reduced level of consciousness.

▶ Worsening or new-onset peripheral oedema or rising jugular venous pressure (JVP).

▶ Low SaO_2.

Red flags: impending respiratory arrest

▶ 'Respiratory alternans' – short-term alternation between using the diaphragm for breathing and using the accessory muscles.

▶ Abdominal paradox – this is a sign of diaphragmatic fatigue. The abdomen moves inwards with each inspiratory effort.

▶ Patient is 'slow to respond' and confused.

▶ SaO_2 markedly reduced.

The priorities for treatment of an AECOPD are:

▷ bronchodilators to relieve breathlessness. These might need to be given in high doses via nebuliser in the short-term

▷ oxygen to correct hypoxaemia

▷ 30 mg prednisolone orally for 7 to 14 days

▷ antibiotics (if the sputum is discoloured).[2]

PULMONARY EMBOLISM

This is an important cause of acute-onset breathlessness. A pulmonary embolism (PE) is a blockage of the arteries in the lung, usually caused by a blood clot that has developed in the major veins of the leg or abdomen, and moved to the lungs along the inferior vena cava. The main cause of venous clots and subsequent PE is immobility, particularly following surgery.

Blockage of the artery causes death of lung tissue (infarction) and a disruption of gas exchange in that area of the lung. The symptoms of a minor embolism are pleuritic pain over the affected area and mild breathlessness. Recurrent minor embolism can lead to pulmonary fibrosis and chronic, progressive breathlessness.

In acute major pulmonary embolism, a large clot causes a blockage of the main pulmonary arteries, depriving the heart of oxygenated blood. Breathlessness is severe, and death can occur within minutes.

Red flags: potential pulmonary embolus

▶ Acute-onset dyspnoea.

▶ Sudden-onset pleuritic pain.

▶ Presence of risk factors for thromboembolism, e.g. trauma or recent surgery, immobility, etc.

Your immediate priorities if you suspect a PE are to make a rapid clinical assessment:

▷ pulse, blood pressure and JVP

▷ respiratory rate and the presence of a pleural rub

▷ SaO_2 (hypoxia is always present with a large PE, but a normal SaO_2 does not exclude a small one.) If the SaO_2 is less than 90 per cent oxygen should be administered

▷ history of risk factors for PE

▷ electrocardiogram (ECG) (to exclude acute myocardial infarction).

All patients with suspected PE will need to be assessed in hospital and will need other tests such as ventilation–perfusion (VQ) scanning, angiography, spiral computerised tomogram (CT) or magnetic resonance imaging (MRI) to confirm a diagnosis.

If PE is likely, once-daily low molecular weight heparin is usually started. If the diagnosis is confirmed anticoagulation will need to be continued. Thrombolysis might also be considered for patients with an acute, major embolism.

PNEUMOTHORAX

Pneumothorax is the presence of air in the pleural space surrounding the lung. The accumulation of air can cause all or part of the lung to collapse, causing acute breathlessness and pleuritic pain. Potential causes of pneumothorax include:

- ▶ spontaneous primary pneumothorax
  - ▷ rupture of a bulla at the lung apex (often occurs in previously fit young adults – mostly tall, thin men)
- ▶ spontaneous secondary pneumothorax
  - ▷ rupture of bulla in patients with existing lung disease (common in patients with COPD – particularly those with bullous emphysema)
- ▶ traumatic pneumothorax
  - ▷ penetrating injury through chest wall
  - ▷ rib fracture (can be caused by coughing in elderly patients)
  - ▷ rupture of trachea or bronchus (deceleration injury in high-speed car crash)
  - ▷ oesophageal rupture (endoscopic procedure or external injury).[3]

Pneumothorax should be considered in any patient presenting with sudden-onset breathlessness and chest pain. Breath sounds will be diminished or absent on the affected side and the diagnosis needs to be confirmed by chest X-ray.

You will need to assess the patient's respiratory status. Check the SaO_2. If this is under 90 per cent an arterial blood gas (ABG) sampling is needed and oxygen should be administered during transfer to hospital.

Tension pneumothorax occurs when the communication between the lung and the pleural space acts like a valve. Air enters the pleural space on inspiration and the valve closes to prevent its escape during expiration. Pressure then builds up, compressing the heart and lungs. This impedes breathing and venous return to the heart.

Tension pneumothorax is a medical emergency. Death from the combined effects of respiratory and circulatory failure can result. Immediate insertion of a chest drain is required.

Red flags: tension pneumothorax

- ▶ Acute and worsening dyspnoea.
- ▶ Absent breath sounds over one hemithorax.
- ▶ Deviated trachea.

Cardiac causes of acute breathlessness

ACUTE LEFT VENTRICULAR FAILURE

Acute left ventricular failure (LVF) is a medical emergency. It causes acute pulmonary oedema and very severe, acute-onset, rapidly worsening breathlessness. A cardinal feature of breathlessness in acute LVF is orthopnoea. The clinical features and risk factors are shown in Table 7.3.

Table 7.3 ○ *Clinical features and risk factors for acute LVF*

Risk factors	Clinical features
Coronary heart disease	Sudden-onset and rapidly increasing dyspnoea
Rheumatic heart disease	Wheezing
Congenital heart disease	Profuse sweating
Hypertension	Anxiety
High altitude	

CARDIAC RHYTHM DISTURBANCE

Cardiac dysrhythmias, as well as causing palpitations, can present with acute breathlessness. Supraventricular tachycardia is a condition characterised by an abnormally fast heart rate (typically 140–180 b.p.m., but up to 300 b.p.m.), which is sustained for a number of hours or days. The symptoms include breathlessness and chest pain.

ACUTE MYOCARDIAL INFARCTION

In some patients (particularly diabetics and the elderly) a myocardial infarction might cause only mild chest pain, which can be confused with 'indigestion', or can be completely painless: the so-called 'silent infarction'. If the infarction disrupts the normal pumping of the heart it can cause acute and severe breathlessness. This can be the main presenting symptom in these patients.

PERICARDITIS

Inflammation of the pericardial sac surrounding the heart leads to the production and accumulation of fluid within the sac. This stops the heart muscle from pumping normally (tamponade). The breathlessness is often associated with chest pain, usually pleuritic in nature.

Other causes of acute breathlessness

SARCOIDOSIS

Sarcoidosis is a multi-system disease caused by an immunological response to an unknown antigen. Patients usually present with distinctive clinical features:

▷ round, red, raised nodules on the shins (erythema nodosum)
▷ joint pain (acute arthritis, swollen ankles)
▷ breathlessness and dry cough.

   Acute sarcoidosis can affect the lungs, causing dyspnoea and a dry cough. These symptoms might follow an upper respiratory tract infection (URTI). Although it often resolves spontaneously within a few weeks, some people (particularly the elderly) develop the chronic form of the disease. This can cause interstitial lung disease and pulmonary fibrosis.[3]

Diabetic ketoacidosis

In uncontrolled diabetes lack of insulin prevents metabolism of glucose to provide energy for physiological processes. The body attempts to compensate with excessive lipid metabolism, which leads to the production of acidic substances (ketones) that accumulate in the blood and give rise to metabolic acidosis. In diabetic ketoacidosis acute breathlessness is a compensatory mechanism aimed at reducing blood acidity.

   As well as breathlessness and metabolic acidosis, the absence of glucose metabolism leads to elevated levels of glucose in the blood. This produces osmotic diuresis, loss of fluids and electrolytes (sodium and potassium), and subsequent dehydration.[4]

   Diabetic ketoacidosis has a number of distinctive clinical features:

▷ nausea and vomiting
▷ a sickly, sweet, fruity smell on the breath ('acid drops')
▷ severe abdominal pain
▷ hyperventilation.

   Ketoacidosis is typically seen in patients with diabetes who:

▷ were previously undiagnosed
▷ have stopped or interrupted their normal insulin therapy, or are under stress from illness.

   Untreated, it can lead to coma and death.

PANIC ATTACKS

Panic attacks can cause acute breathlessness by activating and perpetuating the body's response to fear. As a natural reaction to fear, the body prepares to fight against danger or flee from it (fight-or-flight response).[5] However, this response can occur very suddenly and at the wrong time, when there is no real danger; this is known as a panic attack.

Panic attacks are often associated with specific psychological triggers, such as phobias, stressful events, or the anticipation of a stressful situation. In some cases, the precipitating factor is not immediately obvious. Panic attacks are fairly common, with one in ten people experiencing an attack at some point in their lives.[6]

The clinical features of a panic attack are:

▷ tachycardia, palpitations
▷ dyspnoea, hyperventilation
▷ chest pain
▷ tightness in the throat and choking sensations
▷ nausea
▷ dizziness
▷ trembling
▷ numbness and tingling
▷ sweating or hot flushes.

Dyspnoea is one of the main symptoms.

Although the physical symptoms of panic are harmless, the experience of having an attack is often very frightening, and can be associated with the feeling that something terrible is about to happen, e.g. a heart attack, collapsing, or even death. Psychological reactions to bodily sensations act to increase the perceived threat, which increases the sense of fear and escalates the symptoms. In many people the fear of feeling out of breath can lead to hyperventilation.

Panic attacks generally subside within minutes, although they can last much longer when accompanied by catastrophic thoughts.[6]

Chronic breathlessness

Respiratory causes of chronic breathlessness

CHRONIC OBSTRUCTIVE PULMONARY DISEASE

COPD is defined as:

a disease characterised by airflow obstruction. The airflow obstruction is usually progressive, not fully reversible and does not change markedly over several months. The disease is predominantly caused by smoking.[2]

The disease processes in COPD cause irreversible airflow obstruction and destruction of alveolar capillary interface, thus interfering with ventilation of the lungs and with gas exchange.

Breathlessness on exertion is a key presenting symptom. Its onset is slow and insidious, and might not be noticed by the patient until he or she has irretrievably lost half of his or her respiratory reserve[7] and is significantly disabled by breathlessness. The overall intensity and duration of symptoms increases with the progression of disease. In the early stages breathlessness might only be experienced on vigorous exertion, but, as lung function declines progressively, breathlessness becomes more chronic and troublesome.

The slowly progressive natural history of COPD is punctuated by exacerbations. These produce an acute worsening of breathlessness and become more severe and disabling as the underlying disease progresses. In about a third of cases, an exacerbation of COPD represents a new respiratory event or complication (e.g. infection, development of peripheral oedema, or pulmonary oedema resulting from co-morbid coronary heart disease), but most exacerbations of COPD have no obvious precipitating cause. Clinical features of acute exacerbations of COPD are:

▷ increased dyspnoea
▷ increased cough and sputum production
▷ sputum purulence.

Increased dyspnoea is the main symptom.[2]

INTERSTITIAL LUNG DISEASE

The conditions that cause airway obstruction are common, but few in number. In contrast, there is an enormous number of causes for interstitial lung disease, but it is rarer.[3,8] Table 7.4 is a by no means exhaustive list.

Table 7.4 ○ **Possible causes of interstitial lung disease**

Idiopathic	Drug induced	Occupational
Cryptogenic fibrosing alveolitis	Antibiotics ▶ nitrofurantoin	Asbestosis
Cryptogenic organising alveolitis	Anti-inflammatory drugs ▶ *aspirin* ▶ *gold* ▶ *penicillamine*	Pneumoconiosis ▶ *coal worker's pneumoconiosis*
Cystic fibrosis	Cancer chemotherapy ▶ *bleomycin* ▶ *busulfan* ▶ *cyclophosphamide* ▶ *methotrexate*	Silicosis
Chronic sarcoidosis	Cardiovascular drugs ▶ *amiodarone* ▶ *tocainide*	Byssinosis ○ *cotton workers*
Systemic lupus erythematosus	Illicit drugs ▶ *heroin* ▶ *methadone* ▶ *crack cocaine*	Hypersensitivity pneumonitis ▶ *farmer's lung* ▶ *mushroom worker's lung* ▶ *grain worker's lung*
Rheumatoid arthritis		
Recurrent multiple pulmonary embolism		
Systemic sclerosis		
Extrinsic allergic alveolitis		

Interstitial lung disease is a term used to describe a range of conditions affecting the alveoli and the interstitium of the lung. They are characterised by a reduction in lung volumes (reduced lung capacity) and a deficiency of gaseous exchange across the alveolar capillary membranes. The clinical features are:

▷ progressive dyspnoea
▷ dry cough
▷ finger clubbing (except sarcoidosis)
▷ cyanosis, respiratory failure, pulmonary hypertension and heart failure in the later stages.

Chronic cryptogenic fibrosing alveolitis and cryptogenic organising alveolitis can lead to lung fibrosis, although the progression of disease in extrinsic allergic alveolitis can be halted by cessation of exposure to the causative antigen. The acute form of sarcoidosis might resolve spontaneously, but the chronic form of the disease can lead to interstitial lung disease, which occasionally progresses to lung fibrosis.

Breathlessness and associated fatigue are key features of interstitial lung disease. Breathlessness might be initially only present on exertion, but in progressive and more severe disease can be a problem at rest as well.

TUMOURS OF THE LUNG AND RESPIRATORY TRACT

Lung cancer is the most common cause of cancer death in the UK, with over 33,000 deaths each year.[9]

Tumours that develop in the bronchial tree often give rise to respiratory symptoms. Breathlessness arises because the presence of a tumour can:

▷ obstruct the airway, leading to partial or complete collapse of the lung
▷ lead the collection of fluid in the pleural space (pleural effusion)
▷ compress surrounding structures (airways and blood vessels).

Tumours in the peripheral regions of the lung are associated with few respiratory symptoms until late in the disease process. Patients may present with generalised symptoms (e.g. weight loss) and/or symptoms of secondary tumours (e.g. in the brain or liver). Lung cancer symptoms often present alongside symptoms of pre-existing chronic lung disease associated with a long smoking history (i.e. COPD).[4]

Non-bronchial respiratory cancers include mesothelioma, interstitial lung tumours (which cause slowly progressive breathlessness), tracheal tumours (which present as rapidly progressive breathlessness) and laryngeal tumours (which are characterised by voice hoarseness and can lead to breathlessness).[4]

CYSTIC FIBROSIS

Cystic fibrosis causes chronic breathlessness by impairing the clearance of mucus and disrupting gaseous exchange. It is an inherited genetic disease affecting around 1 in 2500 live births in the UK. The failure of chloride transport in the membrane of epithelial cells affects all the mucus-producing glands of the body, increasing the viscosity of the mucus. This leads to the copious production and accumulation of secretions. Glands in the lungs, pancreas, intestine and other organs become clogged with mucus, and are unable to function normally. Cystic fibrosis is also associated with liver problems, chronic malabsorption and infertility.

Impaired mucociliary clearance of the mucosa in the bronchi leads to repeated cycles of bacterial infection and inflammation, and subsequent airway obstruction. Although most cases are diagnosed in early childhood, some cases resemble asthma that responds poorly to treatment, and the diagnosis can be missed. Some patients are not diagnosed until early or even middle adult life.

In older children and adults, cystic fibrosis eventually leads to bronchiectasis and respiratory failure. The number of patients surviving into adulthood is increasing due to improved management of the disease.

Cardiac causes of chronic breathlessness

HEART FAILURE

The National Institute for Health and Clinical Excellence (NICE) describes heart failure as:

a complex syndrome that can result from any structural or functional cardiac disorder that impairs the ability of the heart to function as a pump to support physiological circulation.[10]

The most common causes of heart failure are coronary heart disease and hypertension, but it can also be caused by rhythm disturbances, valve disease and cardiomyopathy.[11, 12] These conditions interfere with the pump mechanism or with the electrical activity of the heart.

The most well understood type of heart failure is left ventricular systolic dysfunction (LVSD). The left ventricle fails to pump effectively during the systolic phase of the cardiac cycle. Diastolic heart failure is where the heart fails to fill properly during the diastolic phase of the cycle. Less is known about this type of failure and how it should be managed.

Failure of the heart to pump effectively produces a drop in blood pressure and the body responds in the same way as it does to a sudden loss of blood:

▷ the renin angiotensin aldosterone system (RAAS) releases renin
▷ renin activates angiotensin, turning it into the weakly active angiotensin I
▷ angiotensin-converting enzyme (ACE) converts angiotensin I to angiotensin II, a powerful vasoconstrictor
▷ angiotensin II also activates aldosterone, which causes retention of sodium and water.

The effect of this activity is to increase the circulating volume of blood and raise the pressure in the circulation.[13]

When the left ventricle fails to pump effectively there is back pressure in the pulmonary veins. The rise in pressure in the pulmonary circulation causes pulmonary oedema. Oedematous lungs are unable to exchange gas efficiently and are stiffer and less elastic. Lying down compounds the problems and worsens the breathlessness.

In summary, heart failure can cause dyspnoea by:

▷ interfering with gas exchange in the lungs
▷ disrupting efficient ventilation of the lungs
▷ reducing the efficiency of the circulation and delivery of oxygen to the tissues.

Other causes of chronic breathlessness

Neurological disease

Neurological problems, such as myasthenia gravis, muscular dystrophy, lower motor neurone disease, Guillain-Barré syndrome and 'burnt out' poliomyelitis can cause weakness of the respiratory muscles and dyspnoea. The breathlessness is accompanied by the symptoms of the underlying neurological problem.

Anaemia

Deficient haemoglobin means that oxygen cannot be efficiently transported to the tissues and the body will be unable to adapt to the increased demand for oxygen that exercise imposes on it. This results in breathlessness on exertion. Severe anaemia can lead to heart failure, which compounds the breathlessness.

Hyperthyroidism

Hyperthyroidism is the term given to an overactive thyroid gland. The condition affects five times as many females as males, with a prevalence of 2–5 per cent in women aged 20–40 years.[4] The causes include:

▷ Graves' disease (an autoimmune disorder that stimulates excessive production of thyroid hormone)
▷ benign tumour
▷ infection of the thyroid gland (thyroiditis)
▷ over-secretion of thyroid-stimulating hormone by the pituitary gland
▷ excess iodine intake from drugs or supplements
▷ cancer (rare).

Over-activity of the thyroid gland increases metabolic rate. The breathing rate is increased, leading to chronic shortness of breath. This can be particularly marked on exertion, e.g. walking, climbing stairs.

Obesity

Being overweight will make you short of breath. Excess fat in the abdomen and on the chest wall restricts the movement of respiratory muscles and reduces the efficiency of lung ventilation. Moving excess weight around also increases the demand for oxygen.

Those who are severely overweight (BMI > 30) are at risk of developing obesity hypoventilation syndrome, also known as Pickwickian syndrome.[14]

Obesity hypoventilation syndrome is a restrictive respiratory disorder characterised by reduced lung volume and ventilation. The diaphragm is raised by increased abdominal contents, fatty deposits limit diaphragmatic and intercostal muscle movement, increased chest wall weight further reduces respiratory movement, and there is often reduced responsiveness to low levels of oxygen in the blood, leading to chronic hypoxaemia and hypercapnia.

Dysfunctional breathing

Dysfunctional breathing patterns

Chronic breathlessness might have a psychological rather than organic cause. Chronic hyperventilation (also known as dysfunctional breathing) is defined by an elevation in the normal resting respiratory rate that persists (continually or intermittently) over long periods of time, most commonly in response to prolonged stress or anxiety.[15, 16] Hyperventilation leads to an imbalance of blood gases in favour of oxygen, reducing the concentration of carbon dioxide. The patient experiences breathlessness and other respiratory symptoms. Chronic hyperventilation also:

▷ reduces the flow of blood to the heart and the brain, resulting in cardiac and neurological symptoms
▷ causes gastrointestinal symptoms as a result of mouth breathing and swallowing air.

The increase in breathing rate in chronic hyperventilation is less marked than that of acute hyperventilation, as experienced during a panic attack.

Patients with chronic hyperventilation are often unaware that they are hyperventilating, and might wrongly attribute their symptoms to organic causes such as heart disease. However, evidence from several studies has shown a link between chronic hyperventilation and respiratory disorders, such as asthma.[17-19] Abnormal breathing patterns in these patients are often related to anxiety about their condition.

The Nijmegen questionnaire is a simple self-completed questionnaire that takes only a few minutes to complete. It can be employed as screening tool. A score of greater than 23 is considered to be suggestive of dysfunctional breathing.

Respondents are asked to ring the score that best describes the frequency with which they experienced the symptoms listed.

Table 7.5 ○ *Nijmegen questionnaire*

Symptom	Never	Seldom	Some-times	Often	Very often
Chest pain	0	1	2	3	4
Feeling tense	0	1	2	3	4
Blurred vision	0	1	2	3	4
Dizziness	0	1	2	3	4
Confusion or loss of touch with reality	0	1	2	3	4
Fast or deep breathing	0	1	2	3	4
Shortness of breath	0	1	2	3	4
Tightness across chest	0	1	2	3	4
Bloated sensation in stomach	0	1	2	3	4
Tingling in fingers and hands	0	1	2	3	4
Difficulty in breathing or taking a deep breath	0	1	2	3	4
Stiffness or cramps in fingers and hands	0	1	2	3	4
Tightness around the mouth	0	1	2	3	4
Cold hands or feet	0	1	2	3	4
Palpitations in the chest	0	1	2	3	4
Anxiety	0	1	2	3	4

Source: reprinted from *Journal of Psychosomatic Research* **29(2)**, J van Dixhoorn, HJ Duivenvoorden, Efficacy of Nijmegen Questionnaire in recognition of the hyperventilation syndrome, pp. 199–206, copyright 1985, with permission from Elsevier.

Cough

Cough is a frequent reason for people to seek medical help. It can be extremely troublesome and can have a significant detrimental effect on quality of life.[20] The BTS has recently published a guideline for the management of cough in adults.[9]

Cough can be a symptom of cardiac, respiratory and gastric problems. It can be dry or productive, and acute or chronic.

ACUTE COUGH

The BTS guideline defines acute cough as lasting less than 3 weeks.

Acute cough is a frequent cause of presentation to primary care and is most commonly associated with viral URTI; 40–50 per cent of people who have an URTI will have a cough as well.[21] Acute cough, because of its relationship with viral URTI, is seasonal with a peak incidence during the winter. Acute cough can also be associated with exposure to irritant fumes and gases. In this case, the eyes and the nose are usually also affected.

In a previously fit person an episode of acute cough is normally a benign and self-limiting problem. Some people experience a 'post-viral' cough for longer than 3 weeks, but this will generally resolve within 5–8 weeks.

You will, however, need to bear in mind that a chronic cough starts with an acute episode and a presentation with acute cough might be a first indication of a more serious condition. In this case, there will usually be a number of other symptoms present that should prompt you to refer for a chest X-ray:

▷ haemoptysis
▷ breathlessness
▷ fever
▷ chest pain
▷ weight loss.

When you see a patient with an acute cough you will need also to consider:

▷ lung cancer
▷ serious infection – pneumonia, tuberculosis
▷ interstitial lung disease
▷ inhaled foreign body.

TRACHEOBRONCHITIS

Tracheobronchitis is an inflammation of the lining of the bronchi and trachea. In otherwise healthy people, acute bronchitis occurs in the winter and is usually caused by an URTI. Organisms such as *Streptococcus pneumoniae* and *Haemophilus influenzae* are frequently responsible. Coughing and wheezing might be accompanied by mild dyspnoea, but symptoms typically improve after 4–8 days.

PNEUMONIA

This is a term given to inflammation of the lung parenchyma (the gas exchange region of the lung) that is caused by infection. The most common type is bronchopneumonia (where infection has spread locally into lung parenchyma surrounding the bronchi and bronchioles). If the inflammation is widespread within an entire lobe of the lung (or more than one lobe), the condition is known as lobar pneumonia.

The classic presenting symptoms of pneumonia are:

▷ cough
▷ purulent sputum
▷ fever
▷ breathlessness.

The cough might be dry to begin with and may progress to become purulent and/or blood stained. In elderly patients fever might be absent and they might present with unexplained mental confusion.

Chronic cough

Chronic cough is defined in the guideline as a cough that lasts more than 8 weeks. It can have a very significant detrimental impact on quality of life.[22] Severe paroxysms of coughing can produce syncope, and stress incontinence associated with coughing can be a major concern, particularly for female patients.

Interestingly, chronic cough is more prevalent in women. Women are thought to have a more sensitive cough reflex than men.[23]

RESPIRATORY CAUSES OF CHRONIC COUGH

Chronic cough is a cardinal symptom of:

▷ asthma syndromes – asthma, cough-variant asthma and eosinophilic bronchitis
▷ COPD
▷ bronchiectasis
▷ lung cancer
▷ chronic rhinosinusitis
▷ interstitial lung disease.

A cough that wakes a patient at night, or is triggered by exercise, is suggestive of asthma. Chronic cough is a prominent symptom in COPD. In bronchiectasis a chronic cough, with production of copious amounts of purulent sputum, is a key feature. Lung cancer might also present with a persistent cough.

Upper-airway problems are a frequent cause of chronic cough. Chronic postnasal drip is associated with 'throat clearing' and is often worse at night, when the patient lies down.

Interstitial lung disease usually presents with dyspnoea, but a chronic dry cough is also a feature.

NON-RESPIRATORY CAUSES OF CHRONIC COUGH

The common non-respiratory causes of chronic cough:

▷ gastro-oesophageal reflux (GOR)
▷ reaction to medication (ACE inhibitor)
▷ upper-airway pathology (rhinitis)
▷ dysfunctional breathing (vocal cord dysfunction or hyperventilation syndrome).

Medical management is aimed at:

▷ appropriate management of underlying lung pathology
▷ management of GOR using proton pump inhibitors, e.g. omeprazole, lansoprazole, esomeprazole
▷ appropriate management of upper-airway pathology (treatment of rhinitis using antihistamine (mixed strength of evidence) or topical corticosteroid
▷ management of dysfunctional breathing (referral to health professional with appropriate training, e.g. respiratory physiotherapist).

Cough suppressants (e.g. codeine phosphate or pholcodine) should be used with caution as they can cause sputum retention that can be harmful for people with bronchiectasis, cystic fibrosis or COPD. There is also a risk of dependence on codeine-based products.

Dyspnoea in end-stage illness

Many patients with end-stage diseases experience chronic breathlessness,[24] including those with:

▷ chronic respiratory disease, i.e. COPD
▷ cardiac disease, i.e. heart failure
▷ neurological disease, i.e. motor neurone disease
▷ respiratory and non-respiratory cancers.

Motor neurone disease is an incurable degenerative disorder. Breath-lessness and cough are caused by respiratory muscle weakness, and most patients die of respiratory failure within 3–4 years of diagnosis.

In advanced malignant disease, breathlessness might be caused by the failure of major organs and systems, such as the heart or liver, or by the secondary cancers within the lung. Cytotoxic cancer treatment, such as radiotherapy and chemotherapy, can also lead to breathlessness through the depletion of red blood cells.

Symptoms are often relieved by the use of short-burst oxygen therapy. Oxygen for use in palliative care can be prescribed by GPs.

Further self-assessment

Causes of breathlessness:

A ▷ Anaemia
B ▷ Asthma
C ▷ Dysfunctional breathing
D ▷ Left ventricular failure
E ▷ Motor neurone disease
F ▷ Obesity
G ▷ Pneumothorax
H ▷ Pulmonary embolus

For each of the following case scenarios consider which one of the above causes of breathlessness is the single most likely diagnosis:

1 ▷ A 47-year-old man is short of breath on exertion. This started one week ago. He has diabetes and hypertension.
2 ▷ A 12 stone 19-year-old man whilst working on a building site suddenly develops severe dyspnoea.

3 ▷ An 18 stone 35-year-old woman on the combined oral contraceptive pill has unilateral chest pain, dyspnoea and has had two
episodes of haemoptysis.

Key ▶ **1D**, **2G**, **3H**.

Further reading

Bourke S J, Brewis R A L. *Lecture Notes on Respiratory Disease* (fifth edn) Oxford:
Blackwell Scientific Publications, 1998.

Kumar P, Clark M. *Clinical Medicine: infective and inflammatory disease* (fourth
edn) Edinburgh: WB Saunders, 1998.

References

1 • British Thoracic Society and Scottish Intercollegiate Guideline Network. *British
Guideline on the Management of Asthma* London: British Thoracic Society, 2008,
www.sign.ac.uk/pdf/sign101.pdf/ [accessed January 2009].

2 • National Collaborating Centre for Chronic Conditions. Chronic obstructive
pulmonary disease: national clinical guideline on management of chronic obstructive
pulmonary disease in adults in primary and secondary care *Thorax* 2004; **59(Suppl. 1)**:
1–232.

3 • Bourke S J, Brewis R A L. *Lecture Notes on Respiratory Disease* (fifth edn) Oxford:
Blackwell Scientific Publications, 1998.

4 • Kumar P, Clark M. *Clinical Medicine: infective and inflammatory disease* (fourth edn)
Edinburgh: WB Saunders, 1998.

5 • Chaitow L, Bradley D, Gilbert C. *Multidisciplinary Approaches to Breathing Pattern
Disorders* London: Churchill Livingstone, 2002.

6 • Westbrook D, Rouf K. *Understanding Panic* Oxford: Warneford Hospital, 1998.

7 • Fletcher C, Peto R. The natural history of chronic airflow obstruction *British Medical
Journal* 1977; **1(6077)**: 1645–8.

8 • Specht N L. Interstitial lung disease. In: R L Wilkins, J R Dexter, P M Gold (eds).
Respiratory Disease: a case study approach to patient care (third edn) Philadelphia: FA Davis Co.,
2007, pp. 316–39.

9 • British Thoracic Society. *The Burden of Lung Disease* London: The British Thoracic
Society, 2006, www.brit-thoracic.org.uk/Portals/0/Library/BTS%20Publications/
burdeon_of_lung_disease2007.pdf [accessed January 2009].

10 • National Collaborating Centre for Chronic Conditions, Royal College of Physicians.
*Chronic Heart Failure: national clinical guidelines for diagnosis and management in primary and
secondary care* London: NICE, 2003, www.nice.org.uk/nicemedia/pdf/Full_HF_Guideline.
pdf [accessed January 2009].

11 • Cowie M R, Wood D A, Coates A J S, *et al*. Incidence and aetiology of heart failure
European Heart Journal 1999; **20**: 421–8.

12 • Fox K F, Cowie M R, Wood D A, *et al.* Coronary artery disease as the cause of incident heart failure in the population *European Heart Journal* 2001; **22**: 228–36.

13 • Cox B. Diagnosing heart failure *Practice Nurse* 23 March 2007: 44–8.

14 • Koenig SM. Pulmonary complications of obesity *American Journal of Medical Science* 2001; **321**: 249–79.

15 • Davis C L. ABC of palliative care: breathlessness, cough and other respiratory problems *British Medical Journal* 1997; **315**: 931–4.

16 • Chaitow L, Bradley D, Gilbert C. *Multidisciplinary Approaches to Breathing Pattern Disorders* London: Churchill Livingstone, 2002.

17 • Carr R. Panic disorder and asthma: causes, effects and research implications *Journal of Psychosomatic Research* 1998; **105**: 137–41.

18 • Carr R, Lehrer P M, Hochron S M, *et al.* Effects of psychological stress on airways impudence in individuals with asthma and panic disorder *Journal of Abnormal Psychology* 1998; **44**: 43–52.

19 • Thomas M, McKinley R K, Freeman E, *et al.* Prevalence of dysfunctional breathing in patients treated for asthma in primary care: a cross sectional survey *British Medical Journal* 2001; **322**: 1098–100.

20 • Birring S S, Prudon B, Carr A J, *et al.* Development of a symptom specific health status measure for patients with chronic cough: Leicester Cough Questionnaire (LCQ) *Thorax* 2003; **58**: 339–43.

21 • Eccles R, Loose I, Jawad M, *et al.* Effects of acetylsalicylic acid on sore throat pain and other pain symptoms associated with acute upper respiratory tract infection *Pain Medicine* 2003; **4**: 118–24.

22 • French C L, Irwin R S, Curley F J, *et al.* Impact of chronic cough on quality of life *Archives of Internal Medicine* 1998; **158**: 1657–61.

23 • Kastelik J A, Thompson R H, Aziz I, *et al.* Sex-related differences in cough reflex sensitivity in patients with chronic cough *American Journal of Respiratory and Critical Care Medicine* 2002; **166**: 961–4.

24 • O'Brien T, Welsh J, Dunn F G. ABC of palliative care: non-malignant conditions *British Medical Journal* 1998; **316**: 286–9.

Chronic obstructive pulmonary disease

8

Rachel Booker and Simon Gregory

Chapter aims

This chapter will consider the causes, diagnosis and management of chronic obstructive pulmonary disease (COPD) from early screening through to end-of-life care.

Learning outcomes

After completing this chapter you will be able to:

▷ discuss the impact of COPD on patients, general practice and the health service
▷ describe the pathological processes and risk factors underlying the development of COPD
▷ identify the common presentations and clinical features of COPD
▷ describe and analyse the means of reaching a diagnosis of COPD
▷ discuss the main clinical problems and describe and analyse methods of managing them.

Initial self-assessment

What is the risk of a smoker developing COPD? (Please select one.)

A ▷ 20%
B ▷ 25%
C ▷ 50%
D ▷ 75%
E ▷ 80%

Key ▶ **B**.

Which of the following factors are thought to explain the disproportionate amount of COPD in lower socioeconomic groups? (More than one might apply.)

A ▷ Crowded housing
B ▷ Genetic predisposition
C ▷ Low birth weight
D ▷ Obesity
E ▷ Poor access to medical care
F ▷ Smoking

Key ▶ **A, C, F.**

Which of the following factors should be considered when selecting an inhaled drug delivery device? (More than one might apply.)

A ▷ Cost
B ▷ Device size
C ▷ Drug type
D ▷ Patient ability
E ▷ Patient preference

Key ▶ **all apply.**

Prevalence

There are 900,000 diagnosed cases of chronic obstructive pulmonary disease (COPD) in the UK and it causes 30,000 deaths every year.[1] The diagnosed prevalence rate is 1.5 per cent. Therefore a GP with an average list size of 2000 patients would have about 30 known cases of COPD; a four-partner practice with 8000 patients would have about 120.

Diagnosed prevalence rates are widely acknowledged to be a gross underestimate and many people with COPD are either undiagnosed or misdiagnosed. The British Lung Foundation has launched the 'Missing Millions' campaign, which contends that 3.7 million Britons have COPD. It advocates the re-testing of all asthma and COPD patients over the age of 35 due to the rate of misdiagnosis. In an 8000-patient practice there are more likely to be between 300 and 360 people with COPD rather than the 120 diagnosed with the condition. In areas of socioeconomic deprivation with high smoking rates the prevalence will be even higher.

Annual GP consultation rates for COPD are at least twice as high as those for angina, and rise with age. One in every eight emergency medical admissions is for COPD: over a million emergency bed days per year. Hospital admissions make up the major share of the costs of treating COPD and up to a third could be avoided by improved primary care management.[2] Such improvements might include use of inhaled medications that have been shown to reduce admissions and the length of stay, such as long-acting anticholinergics or long-acting beta-agonists, pulmonary rehabilitation and active case management by GPs, community matrons or respiratory out-reach teams.

COPD disables, often for many years, before it kills. It impacts on every aspect of a patient's life. Forty-four per cent of COPD patients are below retirement age.[3] Many will have to take time off work or give up work early. Progressive disability causes financial hardship, social isolation and rela-tionship problems, loss of role and self-esteem, and depression.

In the spring of 2009 the NHS in England will release a National Clini-cal Strategy for COPD that will address many of the concerns and finally give COPD the priority that is needed to improve the lives of the millions of sufferers. This will address the lack of awareness of COPD and focus on the undiagnosed or inaccurately classified, as well as addressing clear care pathways for those diagnosed.

The recommendations include: (1) developing a strategy to identify undiagnosed or misdiagnosed cases of COPD; (2) improving the accuracy of diagnosis; (3) improving support and information for patients and their carers; (4) ensuring that people living with COPD are properly cared for and encouraged to manage their condition; (5) establishing 'managed clini-cal networks' to ensure that everyone involved in caring of someone with COPD, from the GP to social services, provides co-ordinated care; (6) ensur-ing that, if someone is admitted to hospital, the time is used effectively to avoid recurrent hospitalisation; (7) using innovative technology to deliver and monitor care.

Key points

▶ 30,000 people die from COPD in the UK every year. Whilst mortality from other causes is falling the rates for COPD continue to rise.

▶ COPD is widely recognised to be under-diagnosed. The true prevalence rate is likely to be at least double the diagnosed prevalence.

▶ The direct annual cost to the NHS for the treatment of COPD is around £500 million. This doubles when indirect costs are taken into account.

▶ COPD is the commonest reason for acute hospital admission and is costly for the NHS.

133

▶ Early diagnosis and appropriate therapy could reduce the impact of this disease, relieving some of the burden on the NHS as well as improving the quality of life of patients.

Pathology and risk factors

Definition

COPD is an umbrella term for a mixture of pathological processes (see Figure 8.1):

▷ emphysema
▷ chronic bronchitis and small-airway disease (chronic bronchiolitis)
▷ asthma.

Figure 8.1 ○ *The spectrum of COPD*

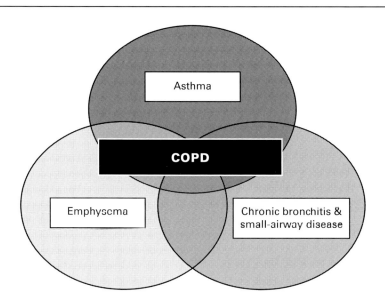

As such it defies clear definition and is therefore described in terms of its physiological impact, airflow obstruction, rather than its pathology:

characterised by airflow obstruction. The airflow obstruction is usually progressive, not fully reversible and does not change markedly over several months. The disease is predominantly caused by smoking.[4]

The clinical presentation is influenced by the balance of these diseases. In practice, most patients exhibit features of all three, but the patient with a major asthmatic component might exhibit some variability of symptoms, for example. If emphysema predominates the patient might be extremely breathless but might not have the chronic productive cough typical of chronic bronchitis and small-airway disease. Although the clinical presentation might be slightly different, the common feature is the chronic, non-variable nature of the condition.

Asthma

Longstanding asthma can result in irreversible remodelling of the airway. The structural changes include:

▷ hypertrophy and hyperplasia of bronchial smooth muscle
▷ deposition of collagen in the basement membrane
▷ fibrosis of the submucosa.

The airway becomes narrowed and distorted, and will no longer dilate fully in response to bronchodilator therapy. Variability and reversibility will be lost.

Early intervention with inhaled corticosteroids might reduce the risk of airway remodelling [5,6] and smoking will increase it.[7] This has clear implications for primary care:

▷ to diagnose asthma promptly
▷ to treat asthma appropriately
▷ to encourage adherence to therapy
▷ to discourage smoking.

Chronic bronchitis

Chronic bronchitis is defined in terms of symptoms:

the production of sputum on most days for at least three months in at least two consecutive years, in the absence of other causes of chronic sputum production.[8]

Many regular smokers have a chronic (smoker's) cough and fit this definition. Chronic bronchitis is not, however, synonymous with COPD. Chronic mucus production might reflect problems in the large, conducting airways where excess mucus does not necessarily cause airflow obstruction. Only some smokers with a 'smoker's cough' will have airflow obstruction – the hallmark of COPD. It is important to remember that not all smokers with chronic cough have COPD, but it is not normal and can be an important marker of early COPD.

Small-airway disease (chronic bronchiolitis)

Exposure to tobacco smoke produces inflammation and recurrent cycles of damage and repair in the small, 2–5 mm airways:

▷ inflammation and oedema
▷ fibrosis
▷ collagen deposition
▷ smooth-muscle hypertrophy.

This permanent remodelling leads to narrowing and distortion of the airway and chronic airflow obstruction.

Cigarette smoke also causes proliferation of goblet cells and mucus plugging. Excess mucus at this level in the bronchial tree cannot be cleared by coughing and might not give rise to chronic sputum production. It can, however, contribute to airflow obstruction, particularly during exacerbations.

Emphysema

Emphysema is defined in terms of pathological and structural changes:

A condition of the lung characterised by abnormal, permanent enlargement of the air spaces distal to the terminal bronchiole, accompanied by destruction of their walls.[8]

Emphysema is, overwhelmingly, smoking related. Tobacco smoke sets up a low-grade inflammation in the terminal bronchioles and alveoli. Increased numbers of inflammatory cells, particularly macrophages and neutrophils, are attracted into the area, and release elastases that destroy lung tissue. Oxidants, released from inflammatory cells and found in cigarette smoke, destroy protective anti-elastases in the lungs. In summary, in susceptible smokers tobacco smoke:

▷ results in inflammation and excessive production of destructive enzymes
▷ increases oxidative stress, escalating inflammation and overwhelming the body's normal protective and repair mechanisms.

The elasticity of normal lung tissue helps maintain the patency of the small airways and produces the driving force to expel air from the alveoli during expiration. Alveolar tissue acts like guy ropes to hold the small, membranous airways open. Loss of these 'guy ropes' produces airway narrowing and collapse (Figure 8.2).

Figure 8.2 ○ ***The 'guy rope' effect***

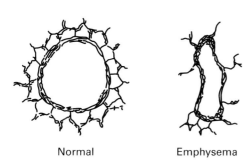

Normal   Emphysema

This is particularly apparent during exercise. Increased respiratory effort produces greater extramural pressure on the unsupported airways. Progressive air trapping during exercise further reduces inspiratory reserve until increased respiratory demand can no longer be met, at which point the patient has to stop (Figure 8.3).

Figure 8.3 ○ ***The effect of increased air trapping in COPD on exercise***

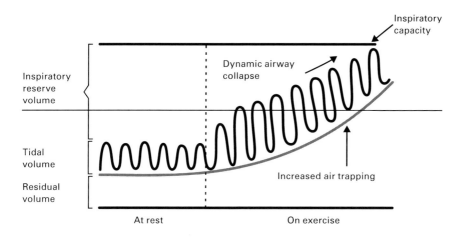

Loss of alveolar capillary interface disrupts gas exchange. Initially an increased respiratory drive can compensate for inefficient gas transfer, but respiratory failure might ensue as the disease progresses.

Long-term oxygen therapy (LTOT) can dramatically improve the life expectancy and quality of life of COPD patients with chronic hypoxia. The key clinical features that will alert you to the need to refer for LTOT are:

▷ moderate or severe airflow obstruction ($FEV_1 < 50$ per cent predicted)
▷ central cyanosis
▷ oxygen saturation at rest of ≤ 92 per cent
▷ peripheral oedema
▷ raised jugular venous pressure (JVP)
▷ polycythaemia.

Oxygen therapy is covered in detail in Chapter 12.

Key points

▶ COPD is a spectrum of diseases including chronic, irreversible asthma, emphysema and chronic bronchitis and small-airway disease.
▶ The clinical picture might vary according to which of these diseases predominates, but the common feature is the slowly progressive, non-variable nature of the symptoms.
▶ Not all smokers with chronic cough have COPD. A 'smoker's cough', however, is not normal and can be an important marker of early COPD.
▶ The small, 2–5 mm generations of airways are 'the silent area' of the lungs. It is not until there is extensive, irreversible damage that symptoms of airflow obstruction become apparent.
▶ Emphysema is, overwhelmingly, smoking related and results in loss of alveolar tissue.
▶ Loss of alveolar tissue has two main effects, airflow obstruction and disruption of gas exchange.

Risk factors

Smoking

This is the major risk factor for COPD; 80–90 per cent of all cases are a direct result of smoking. Seminal work from the 1970s demonstrated that around 20 per cent of smokers are at risk of an accelerated decline of FEV_1[9] (Figure 8.4). Recent work suggests that the absolute risk of a continuing smoker developing COPD is at least 25 per cent [10] and might be higher.

Figure 8.4 ○ *Influence of smoking on decline of FEV[1]*

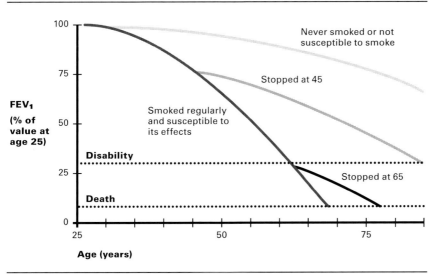

Source: Fletcher C, Peto R. The natural history of chronic airflow obstruction *British Medical Journal* 1977; **1**: 1645–8. Reproduced with permission from the BMJ Publishing Group.

Cigarette exposure, and therefore COPD risk, is conventionally calculated in 'pack years'. Smoking 20 cigarettes a day (a pack) for one year is one pack year, 40 a day for a year equates to two pack years, 60 a day for a year is three pack years, and so on. A significant risk for COPD is a pack year history of 20 or more.

Pack years can be calculated as follows:

number smoked per day × number of years smoked / 20

For example:

40 cigarettes per day for 30 years = 40 × 30 / 20 = 60 pack years

Smoking cessation does not restore lost lung function, but will slow the rate of decline to that of a non-smoker or non-susceptible smoker. Worthwhile salvage of lung function can occur at any stage of the process.

Gender, age and socioeconomic deprivation

Historically the prevalence of COPD has been higher in males than females. However, smoking rates in women have increased since the middle of the last century and the prevalence of COPD in women has risen. In the Western world rates of COPD in women are predicted to exceed those of men in the next decade. A recent meta-analysis suggests that susceptible female smokers experience a greater rate of FEV_1 decline than their male counterparts.[11]

The slowly progressive nature of COPD means that it affects older people. Symptomatic COPD is rare under the age of 35 years and most people are diagnosed in late middle age.

COPD disproportionately affects lower socioeconomic groups. Smoking rates are higher in these groups, but this is not thought to be the only factor involved.

▷ Low birth weight is closely associated with socioeconomic deprivation and is an independent risk factor for reduced lung function in adult life.[12]
▷ Substandard, crowded housing and maternal smoking are related to socioeconomic deprivation and both increase the risk of recurrent lower respiratory tract infection in childhood and reduced FEV_1 in adult life.
▷ A low dietary intake of antioxidant vitamins is associated with decreased lung function. Diets tend to be poorer and lacking in fresh fruit and vegetables, the main source of these vitamins, in socioeconomically deprived groups.
▷ People from these groups are more likely to work in dusty and dirty working environments.

These socioeconomic factors well illustrate the GP's need to provide comprehensive care and to ensure a holistic approach. Simply treating the index patient with COPD is unlikely to be sufficient. In addition to discussion of the disease, advocating quitting smoking and advice on diet and exercise there might be a need to consider other members of the family. This may be about the impact of the patient's disability on them or about health promotion seeking to prevent them also suffering from COPD in the future.

Occupation

Exposure to some occupational irritants is associated with an increased risk of COPD (see Table 8.1).

Table 8.1 ○ **Occupation and COPD**

Occupation	Irritant
Coal miner	Coal dust
Construction worker	Mineral and organic and inorganic dust
Farmer	Organic dust and endotoxins
Welder	Inorganic fumes

In general, occupational exposure is additive to the effects of smoking in an individual. It is, however, important to remember that occupational asthma can result in severe, fixed airflow obstruction indistinguishable from COPD if it is not diagnosed quickly and the individual removed from exposure to the occupational trigger.

Familial and genetic factors

It is not known why some smokers are susceptible to COPD and others are not, and there appears to be a familial tendency to develop the disease, even in families without alpha 1 antitrypsin deficiency. It is thought that genetic and familial factors are involved in determining an individual's susceptibility to cigarette smoke.

Inherited deficiency of alpha 1 antitrypsin, a protective anti-elastase, causes severe emphysema at an early age. Young patients, particularly if they also have a strong family history, should be referred for specialist assessment. Alpha 1 antitrypsin deficiency is, however, rare.

Key points

▶ Smoking is the most important risk factor for COPD. At least 20 per cent of smokers are at risk.

▶ The prevalence rate of COPD in women is expected to overtake men in the next decade. More women now die of COPD than breast cancer.[13]

▶ COPD is more common in socioeconomically deprived groups and prevalence increases with age.

▶ Occupational exposure to organic and inorganic dusts and fumes is a risk factor for COPD, but generally amplifies the effect of personal smoking.

▶ Familial and genetic factors are probably involved in determining an individual's susceptibility to COPD.

Presentation and diagnosis

Presentation

Shortness of breath on exertion is a common presenting symptom but patients adapt to slowly progressive breathlessness. Symptoms are either ignored or attributed to increasing age and general lack of fitness. Twenty-three per cent of respondents to a British Lung Foundation survey [14] had delayed seeing their GP for as much as 10 years after first noticing symptoms. Patients often do not complain of breathlessness until they have lost half of their respiratory reserve, that is, their spare lung capacity, and have moderate to severe disease.

Patients might present with other symptoms before they complain of breathlessness. It should be suspected in any patient over the age of 35 years who has been exposed to a risk factor (usually smoking) and who presents with one or more of:

▷ exertional breathlessness
▷ chronic cough
▷ regular sputum production
▷ frequent winter bronchitis
▷ wheeze.[4]

Obstructive airways disease is common and asthma is an important differential diagnosis to exclude. There are some key features in the history that can help differentiate between these two conditions (see Table 8.2).

Table 8.2 ○ *Differentiating features of asthma and COPD*

	Asthma	COPD
Current or ex smoker	Possibly	Nearly all. 20+ pack years
Age of onset of symptoms	Any age. Often history of childhood wheeze	Rarely under 35 yrs
Chronic productive cough	Rare, except during exacerbations	Common
Breathlessness	Variable	Persistent, non-variable and progressive
Nocturnal waking with breathlessness, cough and/or wheeze	Common. Often a prominent feature	Uncommon
Significant diurnal or day-to-day variation in symptoms	Key feature	Uncommon
Positive family or personal history of atopic disease	Common	Rarely

Recent work has focused on methods of detecting and screening people with early, pre-symptomatic COPD in primary care. The focus is on screening at an early stage. It has been shown that focusing on smokers with a chronic cough is an effective approach. Smokers over 60 with a chronic cough had a 48 per cent chance of having obstructive airways. Even using 40 as the age limit combined with smoking history and chronic cough yielded a 25 per

---

Box 8.1 ○ **_Clinical signs that might be present in moderate and severe COPD_**

Hyperinflation of the lungs

▶ A barrel-shaped chest.
▶ Reduced crico-sternal distance.
▶ On percussing the chest, downward displacement of the upper border of the liver and/or reduced cardiac dullness.
▶ Quiet breath sounds or wheeze on auscultation.

Increased work of breathing

▶ Use of accessory muscles of respiration.
▶ Paradoxical movement of the lower ribs.

Respiratory failure and cor pulmonale

▶ Central cyanosis.
▶ Peripheral oedema.
▶ Raised JVP.

Systemic involvement

▶ Weight loss or cachexia.

---

cent chance of the patient having obstruction.[15] Furthermore, question-naires are an effective approach to such screening.[16] Amongst those with a smoking history the following are strong predictors of COPD: increasing age; cough; dyspnoea on exertion; and daily wheezing.[17]

Clinical signs are usually absent in early disease and are not always con-sistently and reliably present in more severe disease (see Box 8.1)

Diagnosis

The diagnosis of COPD is dependent on:

▷ a thorough clinical history
▷ confirmation of the presence of airflow obstruction with a spirometer.

SPIROMETRY

Spirometry is the only accurate means of measuring and quantifying air-flow obstruction in COPD and is essential for making a confident diagnosis. Measurement of peak expiratory flow alone is insufficiently sensitive to detect airflow obstruction in early COPD and can significantly underesti-mate the degree of airflow obstruction in more severe disease.

Spirometers are now widely available in primary care settings. The person-nel responsible for recording the measurements and interpreting them need to be adequately trained and, preferably, certified as competent.

Practical points

▶ The spirometer must be regularly cleaned and properly serviced and maintained.

▶ Calibration must be checked on a daily basis with a calibration syringe.

▶ Spirometry should be performed when the patient is clinically stable, not during an exacerbation of his or her symptoms.

▶ Height must be measured accurately, without shoes.

▶ You need to record a minimum of three relaxed and three forced expiratory manœuvres with the patient sitting upright, well supported and in a chair.

▶ The efforts need to be technically acceptable (i.e. for forced manœuvres the patient must have made a maximum effort from the start, without hesitation or coughing and blown to maximum expiration).

▶ Efforts need to be reproducible (i.e. the best two recordings of FEV_1 and FVC from the three technically acceptable efforts must be within 5 per cent or 100 ml of each other).

▶ The patient can make up to eight forced manœuvres in a single session in order to achieve three technically acceptable and reproducible results.

▶ For diagnostic reversibility testing the patient should be instructed to withhold bronchodilators prior to the test.

▶ Some spirometry software will store spirometry results in the patient database. If this is not available results and graphs of the forced manœuvres must be filed with the patient's records. Some print-outs fade and will need to be photocopied and stored, or scanned into the record.

Table 8.3 ○ **Normal and abnormal spirometry**

	Normal	Obstruction	Severe obstruction	Restriction
VC	Same as or less than FVC	Same as or greater than FVC	Greater than FVC	Same as or less than FVC
FVC	>80% of reference value	>80% of reference value	<80% of reference value	<80% of reference value
FEV_1	>80% of reference value	<80% of reference value	<80% of reference value	<80% of reference value
FEV_1/FVC, FEV_1/VC or $FEV_1\%$	Approximately 0.75 (75%)	<0.7 (<70%)	<0.7 (<70%)	0.75–0.85 or higher (75–85% or higher)

Graphical representations of the forced expiratory manœuvres must also be checked to ensure that the results are technically acceptable and in agreement with the parameters of lung function.

Spirometry recordings compatible with a diagnosis of COPD are:

▷ an FEV_1 less than 80 per cent of the reference value for an individual of that age, gender, race and height
▷ an FEV_1 / FVC ratio of less than 0.7 (70 per cent).

REVERSIBILITY TESTING

Reversibility testing can be helpful in distinguishing between asthma and COPD where the history is unclear (Table 8.4). Airflow obstruction in COPD is largely irreversible and the lung function cannot be returned to normal. However, some patients with COPD will demonstrate a degree of reversibility, and reversibility testing can therefore be confusing. The NICE guideline does not recommend it as routine.[4] The Quality and Outcomes Framework (QOF) no longer specifies reversibility testing *per se*, but does ask for post-bronchodilator spirometry. In all cases the clinical history, presentation and results of reversibility testing need to be considered together before reaching a diagnosis.

The long-term therapeutic response to bronchodilators and corticosteroids cannot be predicted from a reversibility test and reversibility testing does not therefore provide any information about which drugs are likely to provide benefit in the long-term.

Excluding alternative diagnoses and co-morbidity

There is a considerable number of diseases that afflict middle-aged smokers and can be confused with or coexist with COPD. The major differential diagnoses that need to be considered are:

▷ asthma
▷ lung cancer
▷ heart failure
▷ anaemia
▷ bronchiectasis.

Table 8.4 ○ *Reversibility testing*

Reversibility test	Dose and administration	Lung function measurement	Response
Beta$_2$-agonist	4 puffs salbutamol or terbutaline via metered-dose inhaler (MDI) and spacer (1 puff at a time) or 2.5–5 mg salbutamol (5–10 mg terbutaline) via nebuliser	Measure FEV$_1$ before and 15–30 minutes after administering beta$_2$-agonist	A large improvement in FEV$_1$ (around 400 ml) is more compatible with asthma than COPD
Anticholinergic	4 puffs ipratropium bromide via MDI and spacer (1 puff at a time) or 250–500 mcg via nebuliser	Measure FEV$_1$ before and 30–45 minutes after administering anticholinergic	Some patients with COPD can demonstrate positive reversibility (improvement in FEV$_1$ of 200 ml *and* 15% from baseline) but the lung function will not return to within normal limits
Combined bronchodilators	Give a combination of both beta$_2$-agonist and anticholinergic at the doses suggested above	Measure FEV$_1$ before and 30–45 minutes after administering combined bronchodilators	
Oral corticosteroids	Give 30 mg oral prednisolone for 14 days	Measure post-bronchodilator FEV$_1$ at the start and end of the course of prednisolone	
Inhaled corticosteroids (in patients who are unable to tolerate oral corticosteroids)	Give 500 mcg of beclometasone b.d. (or equivalent) for 6–12 weeks	Measure post-bronchodilator FEV$_1$ at the start and end of the course of inhaled corticosteroids	

Chest X-ray

At the time of initial presentation all patients should have a chest X-ray to help rule out other pathology. Chest X-rays are helpful but do have limitations:

▷ most, but not all, lung cancers will be visible on X-ray by the time they give rise to symptoms. If there is any doubt patients must be rapidly referred for bronchoscopy

▷ hyperinflation ('emphysematous changes') and flattening of the diaphragm on a chest X-ray can support a diagnosis of COPD, but these findings are not specific. Hyperinflation can also be seen in uncontrolled asthma

▷ bronchiectasis is often not visible on a chest X-ray. If this is suspected the patient will need referral for high-resolution computerised tomography (HRCT)

▷ chest X-ray can be helpful in identifying possible heart failure but is not diagnostic.

ECG and echocardiography

Patients with a history of cardiovascular disease, hypertension or diabetes will require particularly careful evaluation. ECG can be helpful, but in cases of diagnostic doubt referral for echocardiography is probably needed. Heart failure and COPD frequently coexist and echocardiography can be very useful in determining which pathology is the major cause of the patient's symptoms.

Full blood count

A full blood count, to rule out anaemia and detect secondary polycythaemia, is also necessary.

Assessment

The post-bronchodilator FEV_1 as a percentage of the reference value is used to classify the severity of airflow obstruction and as a guide to therapeutic approaches (Table 8.5).

Table 8.5 ○ *Classification of the severity of airflow obstruction*[4]

FEV$_1$ as a % of reference value	Severity of airflow obstruction
50–79%	Mild
30–49%	Moderate
<30%	Severe

It is, however, important to remember that classification of the severity of COPD is dependent on other factors, as well as the FEV_1. Mild airflow obstruction can be associated with significant disability and vice versa. Assessment of the severity of COPD should also take into account:

▷ the degree of breathlessness
▷ the patient's health status
▷ their exercise capacity
▷ the body mass index (BMI)
▷ the presence of complications, such as cor pulmonale.

As well as assessing the impact of COPD on lung function it is important to also assess the impact it is having on the patient's ability to function (disability) and on his or her general quality of life (health status).

There are several questionnaires designed to measure these aspects but they were designed as research tools and many are unsuitable for everyday use in primary care.

The NICE guideline recommends the use of the Medical Research Council's dyspnoea score to assess disability (Table 8.6). This is quick, simple and can be Read coded. It is a useful guide to disease progression and appropriate therapy, but less useful as a means of assessing therapeutic response.

Table 8.6 ○ *Medical Research Council dyspnoea score*

Grade	Degree of breathlessness related to activities
1	Not troubled by breathlessness except on strenuous exercise
2	Short of breath when hurrying or walking up a slight hill
3	Walks slower than contemporaries on level ground because of breathlessness, or has to stop for breath when walking at own pace
4	Stops for breath after walking about 100 m or after a few minutes on level ground
5	Too breathless to leave the house, or breathless when dressing or undressing

Source: The National Collaborating Centre for Chronic Conditions. Chronic obstructive pulmonary disease: national clinical guideline on management of chronic obstructive pulmonary disease in adults in primary and secondary care *Thorax* 2004; **59 (Suppl. 1)**. Reproduced with permission from the BMJ Publishing Group.

Many patients with COPD will lack self-esteem and will feel a 'burden' to their relatives. Enquiry should be made about:

▷ how fatigued they feel
▷ whether they feel anxious or depressed
▷ whether they feel in control of their breathlessness.

Clinical depression is common in COPD. Assessing a COPD patient for anxiety and depression is important since this is amenable to treatment and will improve his or her overall quality of life and reduce his or her health service utilisation. GPs and their teams are encouraged as part of the GMS QOF to screen for depression using two validated questions:

▷ During the last month, have you often been bothered by feeling down, depressed or hopeless?
▷ During the last month, have you often been bothered by having little interest or pleasure in doing things?

If the answer to either of these is affirmative then formalised depression screening is indicated.

Key points

▶ COPD should be suspected in any patient over the age of 35 years who has been exposed to a risk factor (usually smoking) and who presents with one or more of:
 ▷ exertional breathlessness
 ▷ chronic cough
 ▷ regular sputum production
 ▷ frequent winter bronchitis
 ▷ wheeze.
▶ The key to early diagnosis is to think of COPD as a possibility! Awareness needs to be raised amongst both the public and health professionals.
▶ The diagnosis of COPD is dependent on:
 ▷ the clinical history
 ▷ confirmation of the presence of airflow obstruction with a spirometer.
▶ Spirometry recordings compatible with a diagnosis of COPD are:
 ▷ an FEV_1 less than 80 per cent of the reference value for an individual of that age, gender, race and height
 ▷ an FEV_1/FVC ratio of less than 0.7 (70 per cent).
▶ The main role of reversibility testing is to distinguish between asthma and COPD where the clinical history is unclear.
▶ Alternative diagnosis needs to be excluded.
▶ The level of disability a patient is experiencing, their quality of life and the presence of depression also need to be assessed.

Management strategies

Preventing disease progression

SMOKING CESSATION

As we have seen, smoking cessation does not restore lost lung function, but it will slow down accelerated lung function decline. Many COPD patients are heavily addicted smokers and find it difficult to stop. There is some evidence to suggest that smokers with COPD are less likely to be able to stop than those without COPD.[18] However, in the recent British Lung Foundation survey of 100 COPD patients [14] 37 per cent stated that their GP had not explained that stopping smoking would slow the progression of their disease and 43 per cent said that their GP did not offer help with smoking cessation now, or in the past. Fewer than half of the respondents understood that smoking had caused their disease.

Where possible make non-judgemental enquiries about a patient's smoking, elicit their motivation to stop and offer support and encouragement at every consultation. Those who express a desire to quit should be advised to use pharmacological aids to cessation, such as nicotine replacement, bupropion or varenicline, and discuss the benefits of this approach with the patient. These aids are more effective if backed up with support. This may be by a practice nurse, an in-house support group or perhaps referral to a specialist smoking cessation service.

Key points

▶ Smoking cessation is the only intervention that can alter the natural history of COPD.

▶ It is never too late to stop and smoking cessation must be actively encouraged at every opportunity.

▶ Smokers motivated to stop should be encouraged to use pharmacological aids to smoking cessation and referral to a specialist smoking cessation service considered.

▶ Don't give up trying to get a COPD patient to stop smoking! You might be surprised how many hardened smokers will give up when they are given consistent advice and help.

Figure 8.5 ○ *The downward spiral of disability in COPD*

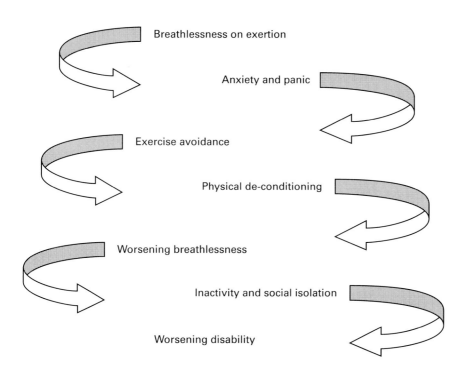

Symptom control

Managing breathlessness

Shortness of breath on exertion is the most common presenting symptom of COPD. Increasingly severe breathlessness is also distressing and frequently leads to exercise avoidance. The patient enters a downward spiral of increasing loss of fitness, progressive disability, and loss of role and self-esteem (Figure 8.5). Eventually normal activities of daily living become difficult or impossible and the patient becomes disabled, dependent, socially isolated and, not infrequently, anxious and depressed.

BRONCHODILATORS

Bronchodilators might produce minimal improvement in lung function (measured in terms of FEV_1) but can reduce breathlessness and improve exercise capacity by reducing hyperinflation and improving respiratory mechanics. They are the cornerstone of drug therapy for COPD.

Both beta$_2$-agonist and anticholinergic bronchodilators can be effective. Anticholinergic bronchodilators may have a particular place as they reduce the increased resting bronchomotor tone thought to be a major component of airflow obstruction in COPD.

Individual responses vary and the drug that gives the most symptomatic benefit needs to be determined by conducting therapeutic trials of 4 to 6 weeks duration and assessing response in terms of symptomatic improvement. The five questions in Box 8.2 [19] are simple and practical.

Box 8.2 ○ *Assessing symptomatic response*

▶ 'Has your treatment made a difference to you?'

▶ 'Is your breathing easier in any way?'

▶ 'Can you do some things now that you couldn't do before, or the same things but faster?'

▶ 'Can you do the same things as before but are now less breathless when you do them?'

▶ 'Has your sleep improved?'

Practical point

Many COPD patients, when initially diagnosed, will have been compensating for breathlessness and will underestimate their symptoms. They are likely to under-medicate if they are asked to take bronchodilators 'as necessary'. In order for them to appreciate the benefit they could gain and to enable you to accurately assess their response it is helpful to ask them to take bronchodilators regularly during a therapeutic trial.

Practical point

Assess post-bronchodilator FEV$_1$ at the end of a therapeutic trial of bronchodilators as well as assessing symptomatic response. This will ensure that you do not miss asthma and will enable confirmation of diagnosis of COPD by post-bronchodilator spirometry, thus claiming the GMS QOF points.

The chronic nature of COPD means that many patients need to take short-acting bronchodilators regularly to control their symptoms. If symptoms remain inadequately controlled (e.g. they are still scoring themselves as 3 on the MRC dyspnoea score) despite regular short-acting bronchodilators and good inhaler technique, you should consider prescribing long-acting bronchodilators.

Long-acting beta$_2$-agonists, salmeterol and formoterol and the long-acting anticholinergic tiotropium, are licensed for use in COPD and provide superior relief of symptoms. They also reduce exacerbation frequency and can improve health status. Their once- or twice-daily dosing regime also makes them more convenient.

There is currently little evidence to suggest which long-acting drug should be employed first. They should be tailored to the patient's symptoms and choice of inhaler device.

Theophyllines are relatively modest bronchodilators. They can provide additional symptom relief for some patients, but their side effect profile and their wide range of interactions make them difficult to use in this group. They are generally a third-line approach.

Inhaled bronchodilators work quicker and produce fewer side effects than oral formulations. Oral bronchodilators are only indicated for the very few patients who cannot, or will not, use inhalers. There are now a very wide range of inhalers to choose from and it would be unusual to be unable to find one that was suitable.

Practical point

When selecting an inhaler device it is important to consider:

▷ where the inhaler will be used (e.g. a large-volume spacer is not suitable for a short-acting bronchodilator if the patient needs to use the inhaler outside his or her home)
▷ which drugs you are going to use (as a rule it is better to use the same inhaler device for all treatments)
▷ your patient's abilities and lifestyle.

COPD patients are older and some might have a degree of cognitive impairment that makes it difficult to learn to use an inhaler. Many are also unable to master the co-ordination necessary to learn to use a pressurised MDI effectively.

As a rule, the simpler and easier the inhaler is to use, and the less frequent the dosing regime, the better.

Key points

▶ Bronchodilators are the cornerstone of drug therapy to relieve symptoms of breathlessness.
▶ Which drug or combination of drugs gives the best symptom relief for

any individual patient needs, to be determined with a therapeutic trial and assessed in terms of symptomatic improvement?

▶ Long-acting beta$_2$-agonists and anticholinergics should be considered for any patient whose symptoms are not adequately controlled with regular short-acting bronchodilators.

▶ Theophyllines might give additional symptomatic relief for some patients but their interactions and side effects have consigned them to third-line therapy.

▶ Inhaler technique must be taught and checked by a person familiar with the device and competent in its use, and a device selected that fits with the patient's lifestyle and abilities.

EXERCISE

The sensation of breathlessness is subjective. There is little correlation between the degree of breathlessness and disability the patient reports and the level of his or her FEV$_1$.

Breathlessness, though distressing, is not intrinsically harmful. Regular exercise to the point of breathlessness is positively beneficial in maintaining lean muscle mass and preventing physical de-conditioning. Regular exercise can also serve to 'desensitise' the patient to the sensation of breathlessness so that he or she is able to do more. It improves a patient's general sense of wellbeing and self-esteem, and reduces the likelihood of social isolation and depression.

All COPD patients should be advised to maintain, and preferably increase, their levels of activity. A regular walk is an ideal way of doing this.

Patients with mild to moderate disease might benefit from referral to an 'Exercise on Prescription' scheme if one is available.

A Borg scale (Box 8.3) can be used to allow patients to assess their own degree of breathlessness during activity. They can be encouraged to exercise between 3 and 5 on this scale. The aim is for them to work up to 20–30 minutes of exercise at this level three or four times a week. The Borg scale must not be used without instructions. For correct use of the scale a user must understand and apply the most up-to-date instructions. (Scales and instructions can be obtained together for a minor fee from Professor Gunnar Borg and Borg Perception. A hospital organisation, medical society, etc. can obtain the authority to distribute the scale with instructions for its patients.)

Box 8.3 ○ *The Borg CR10 scale*® [21-23]

0	Nothing at all	
0.3		
0.5	Extremely weak	Just noticeable
0.7		
1	Very weak	
1.5		
2	Weak	Light
2.5		
3	Moderate	
4		
5	Strong	Heavy
6		
7	Very strong	
8		
9		
10	**Extremely strong**	**'Maximal'**
11		
⇗		
●	Absolute maximum	Highest possible

The Borg CR10 scale® © Gunnar Borg, 1982, 1998, 2004

Source: Borg CR10 scale ® and © Borg Perception. For basic information about scale construction, metric properties, correct administration, etc. it is necessary to read Borg, G. *Borg's Perceived Exertion and Pain Scales.* Champaign, IL, USA and Leeds, UK: Human Kinetics, 1998. *The Borg CR Scales® Folder: methods for measuring intensity of experience* Hasselby, Sweden: Borg Perception, 2004, 2008, can be obtained, with separate copies of scales and instructions, from Borg Perception, Gunnar Borg, Rädisvägen 124, S-165 73 Hässelby, Sweden. E-mail: borgperception@telia.com.

Pulmonary rehabilitation

Pulmonary rehabilitation programmes are becoming more widely available and accessible. Patients who score themselves as 3 or more on the MRC dyspnoea score should be considered for referral to a rehabilitation programme.

Pulmonary rehabilitation is an evidence-based multidisciplinary programme. Access to these programmes is still limited despite strong evidence of their cost-effectiveness. Programmes might be provided on an outpatient basis or in the community. Exercise training is the cornerstone of pulmonary rehabilitation. Other components include disease education, dietary education and psycho-social education.

Managing chronic cough and sputum

Chronic cough and sputum can be debilitating and embarrassing, and may promote social isolation. A therapeutic trial of mucolytics, e.g. carbocisteine or mecysteine, should be considered, and treatment continued if there is an improvement in the symptoms.

Mucolytics might also reduce exacerbation frequency.[20] It can also be useful to teach patients techniques to aid sputum clearance such as huffing. Physiotherapists can usefully teach this as part of a pulmonary rehabilitation programme.

Referral

Diagnosing COPD is not always straightforward and management might be complicated. Referral for a specialist opinion might be appropriate at any stage, not just for those patients most severely disabled.

Referral should be considered in the following circumstances:

▷ the diagnosis is uncertain
▷ the patient is under 40 years
▷ there is a strong family history of COPD or alpha 1 antitrypsin deficiency
▷ the patient requests a second opinion
▷ the patient presents with severe COPD
▷ the FEV_1 is declining rapidly
▷ symptoms are disproportionate to the lung function deficit
▷ infective episodes are frequent
▷ haemoptysis
▷ at the onset of cor pulmonale
▷ assessment for oxygen therapy is indicated
▷ long-term nebulised bronchodilators are being considered.

Acute exacerbations of COPD

Acute exacerbations of COPD (AECOPD) are described as an acute worsening of respiratory symptoms associated with a variable degree of physiological deterioration.[24] There is a change in the patient's cough, dyspnoea and sputum production that exceeds his or her normal variation. These exacerbations are inflammatory in nature and studies have shown increased inflammatory markers. Raised C-reactive protein has been shown to occur

---

Box 8.4 ○ *The most common pathogens associated with AECOPD*[25]

Viruses

▶ Rhinovirus.
▶ Coronavirus.
▶ Influenza.
▶ Parainfluenza.
▶ Adenovirus.
▶ Respiratory syncytial virus.

Bacteria

▶ *Haemophilus influenzae.*
▶ *Moraxella catarrhalis.*
▶ *Streptococcus pneumoniae.*
▶ *Pseudomonas aeruginosa.*

---

in AECOPD but this is not sufficiently specific or sensitive for clinical use, though it may aid research into exacerbations. AECOPD are complex interactions of patient, respiratory viruses, airway bacteria and environmental pollution producing increased inflammation.[25] Box 8.4 shows the most common pathogens associated with AECOPD. Viral upper respiratory tract infections (URTI) commonly trigger exacerbation, especially in the winter months. The role of bacteria is less clear as those organisms present during exacerbations are the same organisms that colonise the airways of COPD patients. Purulent sputum has been regarded as a marker of bacterial infection and studies show a greater success rate if antibiotics are used to treat exacerbations than not.[26]

Mild exacerbations might be self-limiting although a change in medication may be required. Exacerbations become both more pronounced and more frequent as the underlying COPD deteriorates. Patients with frequent exacerbations have worse quality of life, increased rates of hospital admission and increased mortality compared with those with infrequent exacerbations.

Prevention of AECOPD

It is logical that reducing exacerbations will improve the patient's quality of life and reduce hospitalisations. This is supported by studies using pharmacological interventions.[27,28] Reducing exacerbations improves patients' quality of life and reduces hospitalisation.

Environmental pollution

A variety of studies has shown increased AECOPD and hospital admissions in relation to higher levels of air pollution. This effect is highest in the winter months. Particular pollutants include ozone, sulphur dioxide, nitrogen oxide and particulates. Measures to reduce environmental pollution are therefore vital if we are to reduce AECOPD.

Vaccination

Pneumococcal and annual influenza vaccination are now recommended for patients with chronic lung disease. Influenza vaccination is well proven to reduce consultations, hospital admissions and mortality. Its use is incentivised by inclusion in the QOF.

Inhaled corticosteroids

The ISOLDE study demonstrated that inhaled corticosteroids (ICS) reduced exacerbation frequency by 25 per cent.[27] Other studies have confirmed the effect on exacerbations, especially in those with severe COPD. This effect is less certain in mild COPD. There is no convincing evidence that ICS reduce the decline in FEV_1.

Long-acting bronchodilators

There is conflicting evidence about the effect of long-acting beta-agonists (LABA) on AECOPD. It is probable that LABAs do reduce exacerbation frequency. The TORCH study showed that salmeterol reduced exacerbation frequency.[29] Long-acting anticholinergic agents have been shown to reduce exacerbations. Compared with patients using ipratropium, tiotropium was shown to reduce exacerbations by 24 per cent.[28] Other studies have been shown to reduce both exacerbation frequency and hospital admissions.

Oral mucolytic agents

Mucolytic drugs such as N-acetylcysteine have been suggested as a means of reducing exacerbations. This remains a controversial area. A Cochrane review suggested a 20 per cent reduction in exacerbations.[30] 'However the consensus view is that the evidence for mucolytics preventing COPD exacerbations is not convincing.'[31]

Managing AECOPD

AECOPD is diagnosed clinically based upon a change in the patient's cough, dyspnoea and sputum production that exceeds their normal variation. If 2 out of 3 of increased dyspnoea, increased sputum volume and a change in sputum colour are present then the patient should be treated as suffering from an AECOPD.

Increased breathlessness is treated with increased doses of short-acting bronchodilators. The choice of delivery method should reflect the patient's condition and ability. Care should be taken not to use an oxygen-driven nebuliser if the patient is hypercapnoeic as this might inhibit their hypoxic drive.[4]

If the symptoms are severe then oral corticosteroids should be used. These are of greatest benefit if started early. The recommended dose is prednisolone 30 mg p.o. for 7 to 14 days. The stopping of steroids should follow the guidelines in the *British National Formulary*. If the patient is receiving frequent courses of prednisolone or otherwise on long-term oral steroids osteoporosis prophylaxis should be initiated unless contraindicated.

If the sputum is purulent, or there are clinical findings consistent with community-acquired pneumonia, or consolidation is shown on chest X-ray, then antibiotics should be initiated. Such initiation should be based on local resistance and guidance. Typically it should be with an aminopenicillin (e.g. amoxicillin), a macrolide (e.g. erythromycin) or a tetracycline (e.g. oxytetracycline). This should be in sufficient dose to achieve tissue penetration and of sufficient duration (e.g. amoxicillin 500 mg t.d.s. for 10 days).

AECOPD is an ideal opportunity for self-care. At-risk patients should be given appropriate self-management advice. They could be taught to respond promptly to exacerbations and have antibiotics and corticosteroids at home. They would then be encouraged to commence oral corticosteroids if they have increased dyspnoea, antibiotics if their sputum is purulent and to adjust their bronchodilators.[4] They would retain the ability to seek assistance if concerned or not improving.

Hospital admission

The decision about whether to treat AECOPD in the community or to admit the patient to hospital is a complex multi-factorial one. This decision involves the GP juggling person-centred care and the needs of the health economy. Such a complex process typifies the GP's holistic approach. Table 8.7 identifies some of the issues that a GP will consider in deciding whether to treat the patient in the community (at home) or to admit him or her to a hospital.

Table 8.7 ○ *Factors to consider when deciding where to treat the patient*

Factor	Treat at home	Treat in hospital
Able to cope at home	Yes	No
Breathlessness	Mild	Severe
General condition	Good	Poor/deteriorating
Level of activity	Good	Poor/confined to bed
Cyanosis	No	Yes
Worsening peripheral oedema	No	Yes
Level of consciousness	Normal	Impaired
Already receiving long-term oxygen therapy	No	Yes
Social circumstances	Good	Living alone/not coping
Acute confusion	No	Yes
Rapid rate of onset	No	Yes
Significant co-morbidity (particularly cardiac disease and insulin-dependent diabetes)	No	Yes
Changes on chest radiograph	No	Present
Arterial pH level	≥7.35	<7.35
Arterial PaO_2	≥7 kPa	<7 kPa

Key points

▶ AECOPD is typified by a worsening of the patient's cough, dyspnoea and sputum production, which might be purulent.
▶ Prevention of exacerbations should occur at a societal level including reduction of air pollution, at an individual level with preventive medication and across the two as with vaccination programmes.
▶ Exacerbations might require treatment with corticosteroids and often antibiotics. This may be part of the patient's own management plan.
▶ The decision whether to admit or treat at home is complex.

Managing the end of life

The ultimate outcome of COPD should other events not intervene is death. This can be frightening for patients and their families. When the condition can be classed as terminal and therefore palliative care is difficult to determine, it is important that the prognosis is discussed with the patient and those he or she wishes to include. Palliation is essential. As with palliative care for malignancies this will include non-pharmacological treatments including relaxation techniques, breathing techniques and counselling. Family therapy may be required.

There might be anxiety. Buspirone can be employed as this does not suppress respiration, although if rapid intervention is required then a benzodiazepine such as diazepam is acceptable. Opiates such as diamorphine can successfully aid breathlessness; a syringe driver can provide a reassuring constant level.

Further self-assessment

A 57-year-old man with severe COPD has had four exacerbations in the last year. For two he was hospitalised. He is currently taking regular salbutamol and ipratropium. He lives alone.

▶ What changes to his medication might you make to improve his quality of life and to reduce his number of exacerbations?
▶ Who else might you involve in his management?
▶ What information would you give him?

Web resources

National Institute for Health and Clinical Excellence (NICE) *Clinical Guideline 12, Chronic Obstructive Pulmonary Disease: management of chronic obstructive pulmonary disease in adults in primary and secondary care* • **www.nice. org.uk/Guidance/CG12** [accessed January 2009].

Global Initiative for Chronic Obstructive Lung Disease (GOLD) guidelines • **www.goldcopd.com** • [accessed January 2009].

SpirXpert (spirometry website) • **www.spirxpert.com** • [accessed January 2009].

Further reading

Bellamy D, Booker R. *Chronic Obstructive Pulmonary Disease in Primary Care* London: Class Publishing, 2004.

Halpin D. *Rapid Reference to COPD* London: Mosby, 2001.

References

1 • British Thoracic Society. *The Burden of Lung Disease* (second edn) London: BTS, 2006, www.brit-thoracic.org.uk/Portals/0/Library/BTS%20Publications/burdeon_of_lung_disease2007.pdf [accessed January 2009].

2 • Pushparajah S, McClellan R, Henry A, *et al.* Use of a chronic disease management programme in COPD to reduce hospital admissions *Chronic Respiratory Disease* 2006; **3**: 187–93.

3 • Britton M. The burden of COPD in the UK: results from the Confronting COPD survey *Respiratory Medicine* 2003; **97(Suppl. C)**: S71–9.

4 • National Institute for Health and Clinical Excellence. *Clinical Guideline 12, Chronic Obstructive Pulmonary Disease: management of chronic obstructive pulmonary disease in adults in primary and secondary care* London: NICE, 2004.

5 • Walters E H, Reid D W, Johns D P, *et al.* Nonpharmacological and pharmacological interventions to prevent or reduce airway remodelling *European Respiratory Journal* 2007; **30**: 574–88.

6 • Bibi H, Feigenbaum D, Hessen M, *et al.* Do current treatment protocols adequately prevent airway remodeling in children with mild intermittent asthma? *Respiratory Medicine* 2006; **100**: 458–62.

7 • Rasmussen F, Robin Taylor D, Flannery E M, *et al.* Risk factors for airway remodeling in asthma manifested by a low postbronchodilator FEV_1/vital capacity ratio *American Journal of Respiratory and Critical Care Medicine* 2002; **165**: 1480–8.

8 • American Thoracic Society. Standards for the diagnosis and care of patients with chronic obstructive pulmonary disease: ATS statement *American Journal of Respiratory and Critical Care Medicine* 1995; **152(5 pt 2)(suppl)**: 77–120.

9 • Fletcher C, Peto R. The natural history of chronic airflow obstruction *British Medical Journal* 1977; **1**: 1645–8.

10 • Løkke A, Fabricius PG, Vestbo J, *et al.* Prevalence of chronic obstructive pulmonary disease in Copenhagen: results from the Copenhagen City Heart Study *Ugeskrift for laeger* 2007; **169(46)**: 3956–60.

11 • Gan W Q, Man S F P, Postma D S, *et al.* Female smokers beyond the perimenopausal period are at increased risk of chronic obstructive pulmonary disease: a systematic review and meta-analysis *Respiratory Research* 2006; **7**: 52.

12 • Barker D J, Godfrey K M, Fall C, *et al.* Relation of birth weight and childhood respiratory infection to adult lung function and death from chronic obstructive airways disease *British Medical Journal* 1991; **303**: 671–5.

13 • National Statistics. Death registrations in England and Wales: 2005, causes *Health Statistics Quarterly* 2006; **30**: 46–55, www.statistics.gov.uk/downloads/theme_health/HSQ30.pdf [accessed January 2009].

14 • British Lung Foundation. *Lost in Translation: bridging the communication gap in COPD* London: British Lung Foundation, 2006.

15 • van Schayck C P, Loozen J M C, Wagena R P, *et al.* Detecting patients at a high risk of developing chronic obstructive pulmonary disease in general practice: cross sectional case finding study *British Medical Journal* 2002; **324**: 1370–4.

16 • Statelis G, Jakobsson P, Molstad S, *et al.* Early detection of COPD in primary care: screening by invitation of smokers aged 40 to 55 years *British Journal of General Practice* 2004; **54**: 201–6.

17 • Freeman D, Nordyke R J, Isonaka S, *et al*. Questions for COPD diagnostic screening in a primary care setting *Respiratory Medicine* 2005; **99**: 1311–18.

18 • Department of Health. *Health Survey for England: health and lifestyle indicators for Strategic Health Authorities 1994–2002* London: DH, 2004.

19 • Jones P W, Quirk F H, Baveystock C M, *et al*. A self-complete measure of health status for chronic airflow limitation. The St George's Respiratory Questionnaire *American Review of Respiratory Disease* 1992; **145**: 1321–7.

20 • Poole P J, Black P N. Oral mucolytic drugs for exacerbations of COPD: systematic review *British Medical Journal* 2001; **322**: 1271–4.

21 • Wilson R C, Jones P W. Long-term reproducibility of Borg scale estimates of breathlessness during exercise *Clinical Science* 1991; **80**: 309–12.

22 • Borg G. *Borg's Perceived Exertion and Pain Scales* Champaign, IL, USA and Leeds, UK: Human Kinetics, 1998.

23 • Borg G. *The Borg CR Scales® Folder: methods for measuring intensity of experience* Hasselby, Sweden: Borg Perception, 2004, 2008.

24 • Seemungal T A R, Donaldson G C, Bhowmik A, *et al*. Time course and recovery of exacerbations in patients with chronic obstructive pulmonary disease *American Journal of Respiratory and Critical Care Medicine* 2000; **161**: 1608–13.

25 • Sapey E, Stockley R A. COPD exacerbations. 2: Aetiology *Thorax* 2006; **61**: 250–8.

26 • Anthonisen N R, Manfred J, Warren C P W, *et al*. Antibiotic therapy in exacerbations of COPD *Annals of Internal Medicine* 1987; **106**: 196–200.

27 • Burge P S, Calverley P M A, Jones P W, *et al*. Randomised, double blind, placebo controlled study of fluticasone propionate in patients with moderate to severe chronic obstructive pulmonary disease: the ISOLDE trial *British Medical Journal* 2000; **320**: 1297–303.

28 • Casaburi R, Mahler D A, Jones P W, *et al*. A long-term evaluation of once daily inhaled tiotropium in COPD *European Respiratory Journal* 2002; **19**: 217–24.

29 • Calverley P, Anderson J A, Bartolome C, *et al*. Salmeterol and fluticasone propionate and survival in COPD *New England Journal of Medicine* 2007; **356**: 775–89.

30 • Poole P J, Black P N. Oral mucolytic drugs for exacerbations of COPD: systematic review *British Medical Journal* 2001; **322**: 1271–4.

31 • Wedzicha J A, Seemungal T A R. COPD exacerbations: defining their cause and prevention *Lancet* 2007; **370**: 786–96.

Lung cancer and mesothelioma

9

Carol Min and John Wiggins

Chapter aims and learning outcomes

▷ To distinguish the different histological types of lung cancer.
▷ To recognise the common presentations of patients with lung cancer.
▷ To recognise who needs further investigation and referral to a specialist.
▷ To gain insight into the investigations involved in the work-up of a patient with suspected cancer.
▷ To gain an understanding of the treatment options in patients with lung cancer and to demonstrate the role of the multidisciplinary team.
▷ To learn about the complications of lung cancer and chemotherapy-related emergencies that might be encountered in general practice, and how to manage them.
▷ To learn how to approach palliation of lung cancer-related symptoms in the community.
▷ To gain an understanding of mesothelioma and its management.
▷ To examine the role of screening in lung cancer.

Initial self-assessment

Answer true/false to the following questions:

Q1)
  A ▷ Lung cancer is the leading cause of death in men and women in England and Wales
  B ▷ The incidence of lung cancer in women is increasing
  C ▷ 10–20 per cent of lung cancers occurs in non-smokers
  D ▷ The average GP will see two cases of lung cancer each year
  E ▷ The high mortality rates in cancer are due to the late presentation of the disease

Answer ▶ **FTTTT**

Q2) The following are causes of finger clubbing:

A ▷ Familial

B ▷ TB

C ▷ COPD

D ▷ Lung cancer

E ▷ Bronchiectasis

Answer ▶ **TFFTT**

Q3) The commonest presenting symptoms of lung cancer are:

A ▷ Chest pain

B ▷ Haemoptysis

C ▷ Shortness of breath

D ▷ Persistent cough/recurrent chest infections

E ▷ Hoarse voice

Answer ▶ **FTFTT**

Q4) The following warrant an urgent chest X-ray:

A ▷ Unexplained chest pain that lasts for more than three weeks

B ▷ Haemoptysis

C ▷ Increased shortness of breath in a patient with COPD, fever and productive cough

D ▷ Cervical lymphadenopathy in a patient with sore throat, fever and runny nose

E ▷ Clubbing in a smoker

Answer ▶ **TTTFT**

Q5) A 60-year-old man presents with shortness of breath. He has smoked 40 cigarettes a day for 40 years. Which of the following are appropriate investigations to be done in a GP surgery?

A ▷ U & Es

B ▷ Chest X-ray

C ▷ ECG

D ▷ Peak flow diary

E ▷ Spirometry

Answer ▶ **FTTTT**

Q6) The same man has a normal PEFR diary and has been waiting 3 weeks to have his chest X-ray. He calls you because he has started coughing up blood and his voice has changed. He has lost 1 stone in weight and feels unwell. What are the next appropriate steps?

A ▷ Put a second request in for a chest X-ray

B ▷ Request an urgent chest X-ray

C ▷ Refer urgently to a respiratory specialist

D ▷ Refer urgently to the medical team on-call in hospital

E ▷ Prescribe antibiotics and arrange to see the patient in 2 weeks' time

Answer ▶ **FTTTF**

Q7) The following are included in the NICE guidelines for lung cancer:

A ▷ A patient who is referred by a GP with suspected lung cancer should be seen by a specialist within 2 weeks

B ▷ The time from GP referral to decision to treat lung cancer is 31 days

C ▷ An urgent chest X-ray requested for suspected lung cancer should be reported within 7 days

D ▷ Lung cancer should be managed solely by a chest physician

E ▷ All patients with increased shortness of breath should be referred to a specialist

Answer ▶ **TTTFF**

Q8) Which of the following statements are true?

A ▷ Small-cell lung cancers represents 20 per cent of all lung cancers

B ▷ Surgery is the mainstay of treatment in small-cell lung cancer

C ▷ Surgical treatment in cancer is dependent on staging

D ▷ Platinum-based chemotherapy is most commonly used in lung cancer

E ▷ The average survival in untreated small-cell lung cancer is six weeks

Answer ▶ **TFTTT**

Q9) A patient with known lung cancer presents to your surgery with increased confusion. What steps would you undertake to help establish a cause?

A ▷ Take a drug history
B ▷ Measure calcium
C ▷ Examine his or her peripheral nervous system
D ▷ Perform fundoscopy
E ▷ Take a detailed history of the confusion

Answer ▶ **TTTTT**

Q10) The above patient is taking neither morphine nor any other drug known to cause confusion. What would be your next step?

A ▷ Take a sample of blood and advise the patient to rest at home
B ▷ Refer urgently to hospital
C ▷ Give a course of augmentin
D ▷ Take blood for calcium level and refer to hospital

Answer ▶ **FTFT**

Q11) A man with small-cell lung cancer comes to you feeling non-specifically unwell. He had chemotherapy 10 days ago. Appropriate actions include:

A ▷ Giving paracetamol
B ▷ Giving a 10-day course of oral antibiotics
C ▷ Referral to hospital for admission
D ▷ Taking the patient's temperature
E ▷ Dipstick his urine

Answer ▶ **FFTTT**

Q12) A 56-year-old woman with lung cancer tells you she is feeling so weak she can hardly walk. She has been falling at home and recalled an episode of back pain that she attributed to sleeping awkwardly. She complains of numbness around her umbilicus and that she has not opened her bowels or passed urine. What are your immediate actions?

A ▷ Give her adequate non-opioid analgesia and tell her to rest at home
B ▷ Give her laxatives and see if things improve
C ▷ Refer her urgently to hospital

D ▷ Digital rectal examination

E ▷ Check for a sensory level

Answer ▶ **FFTTT**

Q13) A 50-year-old smoker complains of a swollen face. On examination, he is plethoric with distended neck veins and visible veins on his chest. He has stridor. What is the next appropriate management?

A ▷ Give antihistamines

B ▷ Organise a routine chest X-ray

C ▷ Urgent referral to hospital

D ▷ Routine referral to chest clinic

Answer ▶ **FFTF**

Q14) Mesothelioma.

A ▷ It is usually caused by asbestos exposure

B ▷ Patients can claim compensation after a diagnosis has been made

C ▷ It responds to chemotherapy

D ▷ It can be removed surgically

E ▷ It has had its peak incidence and is now on the decline

Answer ▶ **TTFFF**

Introduction

How common is lung cancer?

Lung cancer is the most common cancer in the world. In the UK it is the commonest cancer in males and the second most common after breast cancer in females. There are between 33,000 and 37,000 new cases diagnosed each year, which accounts for 1 in 7 of all new cancer cases. The disease is diagnosed more frequently in men but the incidence in females is increasingly rapidly. The peak incidence is between the ages 70–79 years of age.[1,2]

What are the risk factors for lung cancer?

By far the biggest culprit is cigarette smoking. Between 80–90 per cent of cases of lung cancer are attributable to smoking. The relative risk of developing lung cancer is proportionate to the number of pack years of smoking, but genetic and perhaps other environmental factors mean that only about 18 per cent of lifetime smokers ever develop the disease. There is also increased risk in non-smokers from both passive smoke and environmental exposure to carcinogenic materials, such as metallic dusts and asbestos.[3,4] There is evidence to show that stopping smoking reduces the likelihood of developing lung cancer, even after a prolonged period of the habit.[5]

What problems face GPs in diagnosing lung cancer?

A GP with an average list size will see only one or two cases of lung cancer each year.[6,7] The main problems in making the diagnosis arise from the wide-ranging and non-specific symptoms with which patients present. These symptoms are easily attributable to other diseases. It is therefore advisable to be wary of new or persistent symptoms that develop in high-risk individuals. These include smokers, those with COPD, those with a previous history of head and neck cancers, and those with a history of asbestos exposure.

What are the different histological types of lung cancer?

Lung cancer is broadly divided into small-cell lung cancer (SCLC) or non-small-cell lung cancer (NSCLC) depending on its histological characteristics. About 20 per cent of lung cancers are small cell and the remainder are NSCLC, which can be further divided into subtypes. These include:

▷ squamous cell, 35–45 per cent
▷ adenocarcinoma, 15 per cent
▷ alveolar cell, 10 per cent in the UK.[1]

Some are very poorly differentiated and difficult to classify; however, such tumours usually behave like NSCLCs.

The classification is important because of the different behaviours for the two cancer types, which in turn dictate treatment options. Thus obtaining accurate histology is extremely important.

SCLCs are almost always disseminated at presentation and are therefore treated with chemotherapy. In patients with non-small-cell tumours, the goal is to achieve complete surgical resection if possible. This will be dependent on the staging of the tumour, and sadly many patients are inoperable at the time of presentation. There is increasing interest in the use of radio-therapy and chemotherapy preoperatively to try and reduce the size of the tumour prior to surgery ('de-bulking' or 'down-staging').

Learning points

▶ Lung cancer is the leading cause of death in men and the second largest cause of death in women in England and Wales.
▶ The incidence is increasing in women.
▶ Passive smoke exposure also increases the risk of lung cancer.
▶ Lung cancer should be suspected in high-risk individuals.
▶ Lung cancer is divided histologically into small-cell and non-small cell types. In the UK squamous-cell carcinoma is the commonest type.

Presentation

What are the common symptoms suggestive of lung cancer?

Patients can present to their GP with a range of symptoms, which are non-specific and can represent both benign and malignant chest disease. Often these symptoms have been present for months before the diagnosis of cancer is made because patients do not associate them with potentially serious disease.[8,9] It is therefore important to take a detailed history and maintain a high index of suspicion in high-risk individuals, recognising 'red flag' symptoms, which should prompt either further investigation or referral to a specialist (Box 9.1).

Box 9.1 ○ *Lung cancer red flags*

▶ Haemoptysis.
▶ Cough.
▶ Dyspnoea.
▶ Weight loss.
▶ Loss of appetite.
▶ Fatigue.
▶ Thoracic or shoulder pain.

Of these, haemoptysis is the most common. Its presence alone has been shown to be present in 20 per of cent cases of lung cancer and should alert you that further investigation is needed.[9] The presence of a second 'red flag' symptom increases that risk further, the next most common symptoms being cough and dyspnoea. Interestingly, when presenting in isolation, neither of these are associated with increased risk of cancer. However, if there is also a second symptom, the risk increases again and investigation is needed.

What are the other clinical features of lung cancer?

Presenting symptoms might result also from both local tumour effects and metastatic spread. There is also a number of well-characterised paraneo-plastic syndromes that have their own individual features, which may not, at first sight, lead to consideration of underlying lung cancer. The GP needs to be aware of them.

Local effects include:

▷ persistent or recurrent chest infections
▷ localised wheeze (both inspiratory and expiratory)
▷ chest pain
▷ hoarse voice (left recurrent laryngeal nerve palsy)
▷ dysphagia
▷ hiccups
▷ pleural effusion
▷ Horner's syndrome (ptosis, meiosis and anhidrosis due to an apical or Pancoast tumour)
▷ unilateral wasting of the small muscles of the hand (Pancoast tumours that invade the sympathetic chain and brachial plexus).

Features of metastatic disease:

▷ cervical or supraclavicular lymphadenopathy
▷ hepatomegaly
▷ bone pain/fractures
▷ neurological signs.

Paraneoplastic syndromes are features that occur as a consequence of cancers.

In small-cell lung cancer:

▷ syndrome of inappropriate anti-diuretic hormone secretion (SIADH) presenting with hyponatraemia and confusion
▷ ectopic ACTH secretion (causing Cushing's syndrome, which might be subtle and present just with biochemical changes)
▷ Eaton–Lambert syndrome (proximal leg weakness, autonomic disturbance and hyporeflexia)
▷ cerebellar syndromes.

In non-small-cell lung cancer:

▷ hypertrophic pulmonary osteoarthropathy.

What should I look for when examining a patient with suspected lung cancer?

As a GP it will only be possible to identify a limited number of features without specialist investigation. Important features to look out for are clubbing, lymphadenopathy and evidence of metastatic spread, e.g. hepatomegaly, pleural effusion or the paraneoplastic syndromes.

What do I do if I suspect one of my patients has lung cancer?

Management of a patient with suspected lung cancer should follow NICE guidelines, which were published in 2005.[10] There might be some local variations, but the core recommendations are:

1) urgent chest radiograph when patients present with:

  ► haemoptysis
  ► any of the following unexplained or persistent (>3 weeks) symptoms or signs:
    ▷ cough
    ▷ chest/shoulder pain
    ▷ shortness of breath
    ▷ weight loss
    ▷ chest signs
    ▷ hoarseness
    ▷ finger clubbing
    ▷ features suggestive of metastases
    ▷ cervical/supraclavicular lymphadenopathy

2) referral to a chest physician if:

  ► the patient has persistent haemoptysis whether smoker or non-smoker aged over 40 years
  ► the patient has a chest radiograph suggestive of cancer
  ► the patient has signs of superior vena cava obstruction or stridor. This warrants emergency referral to hospital
  ► the patient is in a high-risk population, i.e. has a smoking history, COPD, previous asbestos exposure and with a history of head and neck cancer. This is especially true if the patient has symptoms which are unexplained or that have changed, even if the chest radiograph is normal

3) patients must be seen under the '2-week rule' in a specialist clinic in order for further investigations to be carried out. In many centres there are fast-track X-ray schemes whereby any chest radiographs suggestive of cancer are referred directly to the chest physicians for further assessment.

Learning points

▶ The symptoms of lung cancer can be non-specific and attributable to benign disease.

▶ Haemoptysis is the commonest presenting symptom in lung cancer and should be referred to a specialist.

▶ An urgent chest X-ray should be requested for anyone with haemoptysis or with other relevant symptoms persistent for more than three weeks.

▶ Referral to a chest physician is also recommended for high-risk individuals with an abnormal chest X-ray and those with new 'red flag' symptoms.

What happens after a patient is referred to a specialist?

Any patient with suspected lung cancer referred by primary care must be seen by a chest physician within 2 weeks. The patient must also be discussed by a multidisciplinary team (MDT) at the clinic. The MDT should also include lung cancer specialist nurses, oncologists, surgeons, radiologists and palliative care specialists. The precise organisation of the 'local' MDT will be governed by local circumstances; it should be linked to a regional cancer network for guidance and peer review.

Once the history and risk factors have been elicited and clinical examination complete, individualised special investigations are arranged after discussion by the MDT.

The key investigations include:

▷ blood tests – full blood count (FBC), electrolytes, liver function test (LFT), clotting, calcium

▷ chest X-ray (if not already performed)

▷ spirometry

▷ a computerised tomography (CT) scan of the chest (see Figure 9.1) • this will give detailed information about the size, location and extent of local invasion of the tumour, if any. It also provides information about lymph node involvement and metastasis. This enables the MDT to stage the cancer and consequently plan optimal management

▷ fibre optic bronchoscopy • this involves passing a small, flexible fibre optic instrument (see Figure 9.2) into the bronchial tree via the upper airway, usually under local anaesthesia and intravenous sedation. The proximal airways can be examined and any abnormality visualised and biopsied using forceps. Samples for cytology can be obtained by brushes or saline washes. This investigation offers a high diagnostic yield for proximal lesions seen on the chest X-ray. It has very low morbidity and negligible mortality

▷ CT-guided percutaneous needle biopsy • this technique allows sampling of peripheral lesions inaccessible to the bronchoscope. It is performed by a radiologist under local anaesthesia using image guidance, generally CT scanning

▷ fine needle aspiration of palpable lymph nodes. Deeper nodes can also be sampled using image guidance

▷ pleural aspiration and biopsy • if a patient presents with a pleural effusion, fluid should be aspirated and a sample sent for cytology; this technique has a high sensitivity but low specificity. A coincidental pleural biopsy can provide tissue for histology, enhancing diagnostic yield; increasingly, this is done thoracoscopically, together with pleurodesis, providing both a diagnostic and therapeutic technique

▷ a positron emission tomography (PET) scan • this uses a labelled isotope of fluorodeoxyglucose (FDG) to help distinguish between benign and malignant lesions shown on CT scans. Malignant tumours are very metabolically active and so will take up more FDG and will therefore show up on the scan (i.e. they are 'hot') whereas benign lesions will not. The technique is valuable in aiding differentiation of benign and malignant lesions; it also enhances assessment of mediastinal lymph node enlargement and the presence of metastases. Local availability of this type of scan is currently variable but, particularly when combined with CT scanning (CT-PET), it is rapidly becoming an essential investigation and will be part of assessment of every patient with lung cancer in the near future

▷ sputum cytology • used mainly when patients are either not fit for or decline invasive diagnostic procedures. Diagnostic value is greatest for proximal lesions but yield is poor in comparison with fibre optic bronchoscopy.

The combination and sequence of investigations chosen will depend on the characteristics of the lesion. The majority of patients will have a staging CT scan and either a bronchoscopy or CT-guided percutaneous biopsy, as a minimum. These investigations and their results should be available for discussion at the MDT 2 weeks after the initial clinic visit.[10]

Figure 9.1 ○ *CT scan of chest showing left-sided mass arising from left hilum with lobar collapse*

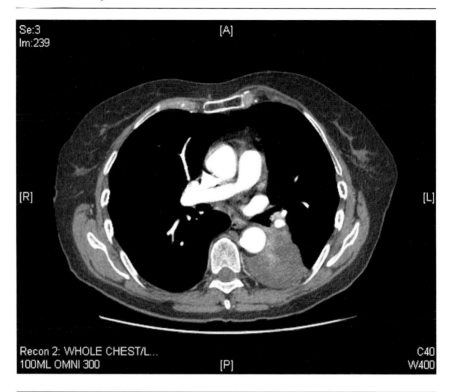

Figure 9.2 ○ *Fibre optic bronchoscope*

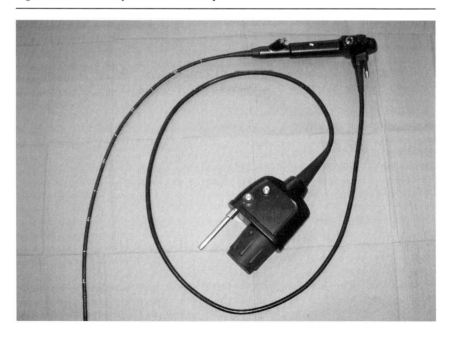

What are the main treatments for lung cancer?

The management is decided by the MDT, which comprises a chest physician, oncologist, surgeon, pathologists, radiologists and specialist nurses. The investigations described above should result in classification of tumour type and its accurate staging, which will guide treatment. Options are surgery, chemotherapy, radiotherapy and active supportive care; the choice depends on individual patient characteristics.

NON-SMALL-CELL LUNG CANCER

The initial goal is to select patients to whom potentially curative surgery can be offered. This implies complete resection of the primary tumour, with little morbidity and an acceptable surgical mortality rate. Such patients will have limited-stage disease (Stage I or II tumours; see BTS guidelines for details of staging),[11, 12] typically a tumour < 3 cm diameter with maximum of one lymph node involved and good performance status, with little or no co-morbidity. This includes age, lung function, cardiovascular risk and nutritional state.[12] Typical surgical mortality for a lobectomy is only 4 per cent and these patients have good outcomes with surgery as a single modality therapy (Stage I: 60–80 per cent 5 year survival, Stage II: 40–50 per cent 5 year survival). Sadly, many patients have advanced disease at presentation and severe cardiac and respiratory disease, precluding any chance of curative surgery.

Some with higher staging might benefit from adjuvant chemotherapy but most remain inoperable. Chemotherapy confers some survival advantage (see Table 9.1) and improvement in quality of life. Current chemotherapy agents for NSCLC are often given in combination and are usually cisplatin-based. The patient should be made fully aware of the side effects of this treatment and that it is not curative, so that informed choice can be made.

Radiotherapy for NSCLC can be given either with curative (radical) or palliative intent. Continuous hyperfractionated accelerated radiotherapy (CHART) is the use of high-dose radiation in an attempt to cure localised NSCLC. It is given in sequential daily doses for up to 4 weeks and has been shown to significantly reduce the relative risk of death by 20–29 per cent compared with conventional radiotherapy and improve survival up to 2 years. It also reduces the risk of metastases.[13, 14]

Low-dose radiotherapy is given as part of palliative care with the emphasis on providing relief of symptoms and improving quality of life. It is useful for controlling the pain from metastases, and controlling haemoptysis and breathlessness.

177

Table 9.1 ○ *Survival rates for non-small-cell lung cancer*

Stage	5-year survival
Ia	80%
Ib	60%
II	40–50%
III	25–30% (surgery alone)
III (with lymph node involvement)	5–10% (radiotherapy alone)
III (with lymph node involvement)	7–17% (radiotherapy and chemotherapy)
IV	2%

SMALL-CELL LUNG CANCER

SCLC is the most aggressive type of lung cancer. At presentation the majority (around 70 per cent) will already have advanced disease. Chemotherapy is the mainstay of treatment. It uses platinum-based agents, given in 3-weekly cycles, typically for six cycles if tolerated. The tumour is re-imaged during treatment to assess response. Initial favourable responses are common but the disease almost always relapses and becomes resistant to further treatment.

Radiotherapy is used in small-cell cancer to consolidate tumours that have already shrunk following chemotherapy and also as prophylaxis against brain metastases.[15]

Prognosis is often worse due to the late presentation of the tumour. For those with limited disease who have had chemotherapy 35–40 per cent will be alive at 2 years. With extensive disease, survival is only between 10 and 12 months. Without treatment, survival is often weeks.

Learning points

▶ Histological confirmation of lung cancer can be obtained by fibre optic bronchoscopy or CT-guided percutaneous biopsy.
▶ Small-cell carcinoma is an aggressive tumour and often presents with advanced disease.
▶ Small-cell carcinoma is treated mainly with chemotherapy.
▶ Non-small-cell carcinoma is treated surgically, where possible.
▶ Too many patients with NSCLC are inoperable at presentation.
▶ Radiotherapy is mainly used to relieve symptoms but can occasionally be given with curative intent.

What are the issues for the GP when the patient is discharged back to the community?

Once there is a diagnosis of lung cancer, a management plan should have already been decided by the lung cancer MDT. There should be close involvement of a lung cancer or palliative care nurse who can act as liaison between the community and secondary care. There are many issues and situations that will be encountered by a GP and the practice. It is important to know how to prepare for and recognise some of the issues, and be able to manage them.

Routine

SYMPTOM CONTROL

There is a range of symptoms that might be encountered; these commonly include pain, breathlessness, nausea (due to the effect of treatment or cancer itself), constipation (secondary to opiates, hypercalcaemia) and depression.

Pain should be controlled using the World Health Organization analgesic ladder starting off with simple paracetamol, i.e.

▶ **step 1** ▷ non-opioids, e.g. paracetamol, NSAIDs
▶ **step 2** ▷ weak opioids, e.g. co-codamol, tramadol
▶ **step 3** ▷ strong opioids, e.g. morphine.

Drug doses can be increased progressively but it must be remembered that often these patients will ultimately require opiates to control their pain and the GP must not be hesitant to prescribe them. Opiates can be given in the form of regular slow-release tablets, patches or as a fast-acting liquid. Oral preparations should be used when possible to minimise discomfort and invasiveness. Other useful agents include anticonvulsants and tricyclic anti-depressants for neuropathic pain, and corticosteroids for reducing oedema or mass effects. Macmillan and palliative care teams have a role here and can advise on analgesia.[16, 17]

Breathlessness is common. Causes can often be elicited from the history and from clinical examination.

Sudden onset is characterised by:

▷ **lobar collapse** • tracheal deviation towards the side of collapse, reduced air entry on the side of collapse, chest pain
▷ **pulmonary embolism** • markedly increased risk in malignancy and might be unsuspected. Often there are no signs on auscultation of chest, and calf swelling or pain might be absent so a high index of suspicion is necessary

▷ **pneumothorax** • pleuritic chest pain, no or reduced air entry on side of pneumothorax, tracheal deviation towards same side.

Gradual onset is characterised by:

▷ **pleural effusion** • stony dullness on percussion, reduced air entry on side of effusion

▷ **enlarging tumour** • difficult to detect clinically but might present with unilateral wheeze or stridor. If stridor is present, the patient needs urgent specialist assessment.

END-STAGE DISEASE

Once this is established, symptom palliation is the goal. Opiates are useful not only as analgesics but also in relieving breathlessness. They also have a calming effect, which contributes to relieving the distress that patients might experience towards the end of life. Oxygen therapy can be arranged at home as part of the palliative care process. Other non-pharmacological therapies include relaxation techniques and psycho-social support.[17]

Nausea is common and can be a result of chemotherapy, the cancer itself or constipation. A variety of anti-emetics are available and oncologists will provide them following chemotherapy. The choice will depend on local protocol. Laxatives have an important role and should always be given when opiates are used because of the almost invariable constipation. If the patient is confused, it is important to check his or her calcium level.

Depression is understandably common and can present in different ways. Self-neglect or 'giving up' might occur. Patients might refuse treatment. Social support is very important and Macmillan nurses are an integral part of patient care and support, along with carers. Antidepressants might be necessary.

Social and palliative care

Patients might need support from social services following diagnosis or treatment for lung cancer. They might be weak or unwell secondary to the cancer itself or following treatment. They might not have family who are able to help care for them. This should be addressed during any inpatient stay and packages of care are usually arranged prior to discharge. This might include carers, meals on wheels or specialist equipment to aid day-to-day care. Other patients might already have a care package and this may need increasing in the community. A number of benefits are available for patients and their carers; local lung cancer nurse specialists play a crucial role in co-ordinating this aspect of care and are an invaluable resource for practitioners in the community. Patients may need input from district nurses, for example dressings, urinary catheter care and management of indwelling venous catheters used for chemotherapy.

There may be a time when patients or their carers need respite, which the GP might be involved in organising.

In those patients who are coming to the end of life, the GP might have to arrange hospice assessment and admission for access to specialist palliative care. Sometimes patients might prefer not to go to a hospice and choose to die at home. This can be a difficult situation for some but it is often possible to provide terminal care at home after full discussion with the patient, family and Macmillan nurses. It is important that the GP is familiar with what is available locally and maintains a low threshold for referral.

The overlap between primary and secondary care for lung cancer patients might vary from area to area. In some instances, the local MDT will continue regular close follow-up throughout the patient's illness. The GP should be aware of local pathways; again the lung cancer nurse specialist plays an important role in maintaining links between the lung cancer MDT and the community.

Oncological emergencies

If a patient with known lung cancer becomes unwell, there are certain diagnoses that warrant emergency admission and GPs need to be aware of these.

These are:

NEUTROPENIC SEPSIS

Typically, this occurs 7–10 days post-chemotherapy as a result of bone marrow suppression. The patient might be either non-specifically unwell or have focal symptoms. They will have temperatures and will ultimately need emergency admission to hospital for intravenous antibiotics, barrier nursing and possibly injections of granulocyte colony stimulation factor to try and replenish the white cell count.

HYPERCALCAEMIA

This might be secondary to either metastatic disease or ectopic parathyroid hormone-related peptide (PTHrP) release secretion, resulting in increased bone resorption leading to hypercalcaemia. Patients might present with nausea, vomiting, confusion, constipation, bone pain and thirst. It is important to measure the calcium level in GP practice if any lung cancer patient develops these symptoms and, if confirmed, prompt admission for intravenous fluids and bisphosphonate treatment if warranted.

SPINAL CORD COMPRESSION

If a patient with known lung cancer presents with leg weakness, back pain, numbness in a dermatomal distribution (a sensory level) and sphincter disturbance (urinary or faecal incontinence or retention) the important differential diagnosis to consider is spinal cord compression. This needs urgent admission to hospital. It occurs in a small proportion of patients with lung cancer but awareness and prompt action is necessary. Another potential diagnosis is brain metastasis but generally this would not cause sphincter disturbance. The patient will need an urgent MRI of the spine and perhaps a CT scan of the head. Treatment includes high-dose steroid treatment, radiotherapy and surgical intervention in selected patients. Surgical decompression together with radiotherapy has been shown to improve outcome in the ability to walk and maintain continence for significantly longer than radiotherapy alone.[18, 19]

SUPERIOR VENA CAVA OBSTRUCTION

Tumours may obstruct the superior vena cava (SVCO) by a direct mass effect or indirectly by compression by enlarged lymph nodes. Clinically, this might manifest itself by facial plethora, distended neck and chest wall veins. Treatment with radiotherapy and chemotherapy might provide relief of obstruction of 60 per cent of NSCLCs and 77 per cent of SCLCs,[20] whilst expandable metallic stent insertion provides rapid revascularisation of the SVC and relieves up to 95 per cent of cases. Steroids can be used in the interim whilst treatment is decided upon, but there are no studies to determine their effectiveness.

Learning points

▶ Symptom control can be achieved using a range of pharmacological and non-pharmacological methods.

▶ Breathlessness can be caused by airway obstruction, lobar collapse, pleural effusions, pulmonary emboli and end-stage lung cancer. Treatment will depend on the cause.

▶ Palliation is an essential part of patient care in the community and should involve an MDT approach (GP, Macmillan nurse, district nurse, palliative care teams, physiotherapists).

▶ The local lung cancer nurse specialist provides a vital link between primary and secondary care.

▶ Oncological emergencies include neutropenic sepsis, spinal cord compression, malignant hypercalcaemia and superior vena cava obstruction.

Mesothelioma

Asbestos exposure causes a variety of intrathoracic diseases. These range from benign (e.g. pleural plaques and pleural thickening) to life threatening (e.g. asbestosis and mesothelioma). It is important that the GP is aware of this distinction, as it is not uncommon for all asbestos-related diseases to be referred to incorrectly as 'asbestosis' by non-specialists.

Mesothelioma is a malignant tumour of the pleura that is almost always caused by asbestos exposure. There is a long lag time between exposure and development of the disease, usually between 20 and 40 years. The incidence has risen progressively over the last decade and is expected to continue to rise until its peak is reached around 2010–15, when it is expected to cause over 2000 deaths annually.

Traditionally those primarily affected have worked in docks, asbestos product manufacture, railway engineering, lagging and construction. However, it is increasingly recognised that many other workers in occupations where asbestos exposure was not immediately obvious are at risk of developing the disease. These include many building workers. Thus a detailed occupational history is crucial in any patient presenting with a relevant symptom, which are typically breathlessness due to a pleural effusion and dull chest wall pain.

It is vital that patients in whom this diagnosis is suspected are referred promptly to the local lung cancer MDT using the '2-week rule'.

Diagnosis is established either using CT scanning and biopsy of the pleura or analysis of aspirated pleural fluid in those with a pleural effusion. The prognosis is dismal and the disease is almost always fatal. Chemotherapy might offer modest survival benefits and there are clinical trials looking at the effectiveness of surgery (extrapleural pneumonectomy, i.e. removal of the lung and pleura on the affected side).[21] It is currently a controversial subject.

Patients with a diagnosis of mesothelioma are entitled to financial compensation and benefits, on which the MDT will have advice. In brief, the patient is entitled to Industrial Injuries Disablement Benefit and can sue a former employer at common law[22] if it can be proved that the patient was negligently exposed to asbestos.

Screening

Screening for lung cancer is controversial. Its value is currently unproven although there is much research ongoing in this area. Earlier studies have shown that screening using chest radiographs and sputum cytology detected tumours at an earlier stage but did not improve overall mortality,[23] probably because of a combination of 'lead-time bias' (i.e. early detection of tumours for which treatment does not alter survival) and 'length-time bias' (i.e. early detection of tumours with an indolent course).

More recent trials using CT scanning to screen high-risk populations have shown that the technique can detect early lesions but many of these proved to be benign. There has been criticism that this then puts patients at unnecessary risk from further examinations and procedures.[24–27] Currently there are ongoing trials, which should clarify whether this is a worthwhile tool.

Learning points

▶ Mesothelioma is caused by asbestos exposure. There is a long delay from exposure to presentation of cancer.
▶ Screening for lung cancer has not been proven to be of use in detection of lung cancer.

Further self-assessment

Answer **true / false** to the following questions.

Q1)
  A ▷ Lung cancer is the leading cause of death in men and women in England and Wales
  B ▷ The incidence of lung cancer in women is increasing
  C ▷ 20 per cent of lung cancers occurs in non-smokers
  D ▷ The average GP will see two cases of lung cancer each year
  E ▷ The high mortality rates in cancer are due to the late presentation of the disease

Answer ▶ **F T T T T**

Q2) The commonest presenting symptoms of lung cancer are:

  A ▷ Chest pain
  B ▷ Haemoptysis

C ▷ Shortness of breath

D ▷ Persistent cough/recurrent chest infections

E ▷ Hoarse voice

Answer ▶ **FTFTT**

Q3) The following warrant an urgent chest X-ray:

A ▷ Unexplained chest pain that lasts for more than 3 weeks

B ▷ Haemoptysis

C ▷ Increased shortness of breath in a patient with COPD, fever and productive cough

D ▷ Cervical lymphadenopathy in a patient with sore throat, fever and runny nose

E ▷ Clubbing in a smoker

Answer ▶ **TTTFT**

Q4) The following are included in the NICE guidelines for lung cancer:

A ▷ A patient with suspected lung cancer who is referred by a GP should be seen by a specialist within 2 weeks

B ▷ The time from GP referral to decision to treat lung cancer is 31 days

C ▷ An urgent chest X-ray requested for lung cancer should be reported within 7 days

D ▷ Lung cancer should be managed by a lung specialist alone

E ▷ All patients with increased shortness of breath should be referred to a specialist

Answer ▶ **TTTFF**

Q5) Which of the following statements are true?

A ▷ Small-cell lung cancers represent 20 per cent of all lung cancers

B ▷ Surgery is the mainstay of treatment in small-cell lung cancer

C ▷ Surgical treatment in cancer is dependent on staging

D ▷ Platinum-based chemotherapy is most commonly used in lung cancer

E ▷ The average survival in untreated small-cell lung cancer is 6 weeks

Answer ▶ **TFTTT**

Q6) A man with small-cell lung cancer comes to you feeling non-specifically unwell. He had chemotherapy 10 days ago. Appropriate actions include:

A ▷ Giving paracetamol
B ▷ Giving a 10-day course of oral antibiotics
C ▷ Referral to hospital for admission
D ▷ Taking the patient's temperature
E ▷ Dipstick his urine

Answer ▶ **F F T T T**

Q7) A 56-year-old woman with lung cancer tells you she is feeling so weak she can hardly walk. She has been falling at home and recalled an episode of back pain, which she attributed to sleeping awkwardly. She complains of numbness around her umbilicus and that she has not opened her bowels or passed urine. What are you immediate actions?

A ▷ Give her adequate non-opioid analgesia and tell her to rest at home
B ▷ Give her laxatives and see if things improve
C ▷ Refer her urgently to hospital
D ▷ Digital rectal examination
E ▷ Check for a sensory level

Answer ▶ **F F T T T**

Q8) A 50-year-old smoker complains of a rash in his face. On examination, he is plethoric with distended neck veins and visible veins on his chest. He has some stridor. What is the next appropriate management?

A ▷ Give antihistamines
B ▷ Organise for a routine chest X-ray
C ▷ Urgent referral to hospital
D ▷ Routine referral to chest clinic

Answer ▶ **F F T F**

Q9) Mesothelioma.

A ▷ Is secondary to asbestos exposure
B ▷ Patients can claim compensation after a diagnosis has been made
C ▷ Responds to chemotherapy
D ▷ Can be removed surgically
E ▷ Has had its peak incidence and is now on the decline

Answer ▶ **T T F F F**

Q10) The following people should be involved in community care of patients with lung cancer:

A ▷ District nurse

B ▷ Lung cancer specialist nurse

C ▷ Physiotherapist

D ▷ Respiratory specialist

E ▷ GP

F ▷ Palliative care team

Answer ▶ **TTTTT**

References

1 • Cancer Research UK, www.cancerresearchuk.org [accessed January 2009].

2 • NHS Information Centre. *National Lung Cancer Audit: key findings about the quality of care for people with lung cancer in England incorporating headline and completeness data for Wales. Report for the audit period 2005* London: NHS Information Centre, 2006.

3 • Hackshaw A K, Law M R, Wald N J. The accumulated evidence on lung cancer and environmental tobacco smoke *British Medical Journal* 1997; **315(7114)**: 980–8.

4 • Wells A J. Lung cancer from passive smoking at work *American Journal of Public Health* 1998; **88(7)**: 1011–12.

5 • Baser S, Shannon V R, Eapen G A, *et al.* Smoking cessation after diagnosis is associated with a beneficial effect on performance status *Chest* 2006; **130(6)**: 1784–90.

6 • Weller D, Campbell C. Early lung cancer detection: the role of primary care *Primary Care Respiratory Journal* 2006; **15**: 323–5.

7 • Hamilton W, Sharp D. Diagnosis of lung cancer in primary care: a structured review *Family Practice* 2004; **21(6)**: 605–11.

8 • Hamilton W, Peters T J, Round A, *et al.* What are the clinical features of lung cancer before the diagnosis is made? A population based case-control study *Thorax* 2005; **60**: 1059–65.

9 • Birring S S, Peake M D. Symptoms and the early diagnosis of lung cancer *Thorax* 2005; **60**: 268–9.

10 • National Institute for Health and Clinical Excellence. *Clinical Guideline 24, Lung Cancer* London: NICE, 2005, www.nice.org.uk/CG024NICEguideline [accessed January 2009].

11 • Chapman S, Robinson G, Stradling J, *et al. Oxford Handbook of Respiratory Medicine* Oxford: Oxford University Press, 2005.

12 • BTS/SCTS. Guidelines on the selection with lung cancer for surgery *Thorax* 2001; **56**: 89–108.

13 • Saunders M, Dische S, Barrett A, *et al.* Continuous, hyperfractionated, accelerated radiotherapy (CHART) versus conventional radiotherapy in non-small cell lung cancer: mature data from the randomised multicentre trial. CHART steering committee *Radiotherapy and Oncology* 1999; **52(2)**: 137–48.

14 • Saunders M, Dische S, Barrett A, *et al*. Continuous, hyperfractionated, accelerated radiotherapy (CHART) versus conventional radiotherapy in non-small cell lung cancer: mature data from the randomised multicentre trial. CHART steering committee *Lancet* 1997; **350(9072)**: 161–5.

15 • Molina JR, Adjei AA, Jett JR. Advances in chemotherapy of non-small cell lung cancer *Chest* 2006; **130(4)**: 1211–19.

16 • Kvale PA, Simoff M, Prakash UBS. Palliative care *Chest* 2003; **123**: 284–311.

17 • Bredin M, Corner J, Krishnasamy M, *et al*. Multicentre randomised controlled trial of nursing intervention for breathlessness in patients with lung cancer *British Medical Journal* 1999; **318(7188)**: 901–4.

18 • National Cancer Institute (US). www.cancer.gov [accessed January 2009]

19 • Patchell RA, Tibbs PA, Regine WF, *et al*. Direct decompressive surgical resection in the treatment of spinal cord compression caused by metastatic cancer: a randomised trial *Lancet* 2005; **366(9486)**: 643–8.

20 • Rowell NP, Gleeson FV. Steroids, radiotherapy, chemotherapy and stents for superior vena caval obstruction in carcinoma of the bronchus *Cochrane Database of Systematic Reviews* 2001, Issue 4. Art. No.: CD001316. DOI: 10.1002/14651858.CD001316.

21 • Treasure T, Tan C, Lang-Lazdunski L, *et al*. The MARS trial: mesothelioma and radical surgery *Interactive Cardiovascular and Thoracic Surgery* 2006; **5**: 58–9.

22 • British Thoracic Society. BTS statement on malignant mesothelioma in the United Kingdom. British Thoracic Society Standards of Care Committee *Thorax* 2001; **56**: 250–65.

23 • Read C, Janes S, George J, *et al*. Early lung cancer: screening and detection *Primary Care Respiratory Journal* 2006; **15**: 332–6.

24 • Silvestri GA, Spiro SG. Carcinoma of the bronchus 60 years later *Thorax* 2006; **61**: 1023–8.

25 • Black C, de Verteuil R, Walker S, *et al*. Population screening for lung cancer using computed tomography, is there evidence of clinical effectiveness? A systemic review of the literature *Thorax* 2007; **62**: 131–8.

26 • McMahon PM, Christiani DC. Computed tomography screening for lung cancer *British Medical Journal* 2007; **334(7588)**: 271.

27 • Spiro SG. Screening for lung cancer: yet another problem *Thorax* 2007; **62**: 105–6.

Occupational lung disorders

10

David Fishwick

Chapter aims

This chapter will cover the main occupational lung disorders, their common causes and presentations, typical early investigations and indications for specialist referral.

Learning outcomes

After reading this chapter, you will be familiar with the common occupational lung disorders, and the approach to diagnosis. Those included are:

▶ asthma and the workplace
  ▷ occupational asthma (OA) due directly to sensitisation
  ▷ asthma aggravated in the workplace
  ▷ acute irritant-induced asthma (AIIA) (formerly termed 'reactive airways dysfunction syndrome')
▶ chronic obstructive pulmonary disease (COPD)
▶ extrinsic allergic alveolitis (hypersensitivity pneumonitis)
▶ pneumoconioses
  ▷ fibrogenic dusts
  ▷ non-fibrogenic dusts
▶ asbestos-related problems
  ▷ pleural plaques
  ▷ pleural thickening and benign pleural effusions
  ▷ asbestosis
▶ malignancy
  ▷ malignant mesothelioma
  ▷ lung cancer
▶ other
  ▷ sick-building syndrome
  ▷ the upper airway.

Finally, various issues including compensation, workability and referral for specialist opinion will be discussed.

Self-assessment

Before reading this chapter we suggest that you consider the following questions. After reading the chapter you might wish to revisit your answers.
▷ What are the clinical features associated with OA? This is asthma due directly to work and due to allergy to a workplace agent.
▷ How would you describe the current risk factors for COPD, and what role does occupation play?
▷ What is the significance of pleural plaques seen on a chest X-ray (CXR) in a patient with no symptoms?
▷ If you diagnose occupational lung disease, who should you tell and what advice should you give the patient?

Introduction

The lungs and the workplace frequently interact. Whilst traditional occupational lung diseases such as certain pneumoconiosis are becoming less common, workplaces are evolving and in certain cases becoming much more complex. Respiratory consultations in primary care are common, and common in people of working age. Not asking about work, and specifically the job and tasks performed, might do the patient a significant disservice. Many patients with lung disease either caused or aggravated by their current or previous work will require more specialist assessment. Delays in identifying such workers will inevitably lead to a delay in removing workers from potentially harmful exposures. The title of a primary care-based editorial sums up the issue well with respect to asthma 'If you want to cure their asthma, ask about their job!'

Asthma and the workplace

Asthma in the workplace is a complex subject, and certain diagnostic issues remain controversial. For the purposes of this chapter, asthma will be dealt with in three separate categories (in practice, there might well be some overlap, and in certain patients an accurate diagnosis will not be possible).

First, and the most important to identify early in primary care, is asthma predominantly caused by exposure at work. This normally implies exposure to an agent or agents capable of causing asthma (asthmagens). Some form of allergic reaction is assumed, although the exact detail for each allergen is not known.

Second, asthma aggravated by the workplace will be briefly considered. This term implies that, whilst at work, a patient with asthma might develop increased symptoms for a number of reasons, but that the workplace exposures do not cause the asthma seen, and neither do they worsen asthma over time.

Third, AIIA will be discussed. This is a specific form of OA normally due directly to a single large exposure to a workplace irritant, normally as part of an accidental spillage or release.

OA due directly to sensitisation

OA due directly to an asthmagen is likely to be responsible for approximately 10–15 per cent of all adult-onset asthma. This figure is remarkably consistent between studies. In other words, one in ten workers with adult-onset asthma have a significant occupational component to their asthma. This fact has clear relevance to preventing disease of the patient and potentially of other co-workers at the same workplace.

CAUSES

Box 10.1 illustrates the common occupations reported to the Surveillance of Work-Related and Occupational Respiratory Disease (SWORD) scheme for OA, as summarised in recent British Occupational Health Research Foundation (BOHRF) OA guidance[1] and in the recent OA standards of care.[2]

COMMON SYMPTOMS

The symptoms of OA are no different from non-OA, namely episodic wheeze, shortness of breath, cough and chest tightness. Typically, they start after a period of exposure with no symptoms (the latent period). The latent period varies, but is usually between a few months and 3 years.

It is the 'work relatedness' of these symptoms that will raise suspicion of an occupational cause. Work-related symptoms normally commence *after* starting work with a particular asthmagen, and are reported by patients to be better on rest days and holidays, worsening on return to work. Various

---

Box 10.1 ○ **Common occupations with OA**

▶ Paint sprayers.
▶ Bakers and pastry makers.
▶ Nurses.
▶ Chemical workers.
▶ Animal handlers.
▶ Welders.
▶ Food-processing workers.
▶ Timber workers.

---

patterns of work relatedness are described, including day-by-day worsening through the working week, with improvement on the first rest day.

Nasal symptoms due to work are also common, and occupational rhinitis is a common forerunner of OA. Indeed, those with allergic mediated occupational rhinitis (common in workers listed in many of the work categories in Box 10.1) are at increased risk of subsequently developing OA in the next year or so. Always ask about job and job tasks in patients with persistent nasal symptoms.

Because OA represents such a substantial proportion of adult-onset asthma, it is essential to ask all adults with (1) possible asthma, (2) new-onset asthma, (3) reappearance of childhood asthma, (4) unexplained deterioration in asthma control or (5) airflow obstruction ($FEV_1 / FVC < 70$ per cent):

1 ▷ What is your current job?
2 ▷ Are your symptoms (e.g. wheeze) the same, better or worse on rest days?
3 ▷ Are your symptoms (e.g. chest tightness) the same, better or worse on holidays?

If patients report being better on rest days or holidays, you have just documented a 'work effect' of their asthma. This group of patients is at much higher risk of OA, and a decision needs to be made whether further investigations are carried out. In current workers, it might be difficult to defend the stance of ignoring this symptom pattern.

INITIAL INVESTIGATIONS

Following routine blood investigations and FEV_1 and FVC, serial measures of peak flow (PEF) should be started as soon as possible. As time passes, obtaining good-quality records might become more difficult (for example, the worker might choose to leave the workplace, or be required to by his or her employer).

Serial PEF should be recorded at least four times a day for four continuous weeks in the first instance. It is best to aim for 2-hourly readings, so that practically at least four good measures per day will be achieved. Suitable record forms can be downloaded from www.occupationalasthma.com, www.hsl.gov.uk/cwh or www.scottishshield.org.

If inhaled medication, including steroids, is required during the period of measurement, doses should be kept constant and as low as possible.

If the worker is currently not exposed, a two-week period of PEF measures can be recorded, and followed by a return to work during which PEF measures are continued. All recordings should be written on a standard pro forma and then entered into suitable software for PEF analysis.

REFERRAL

Workers with asthma symptoms worse at work or improving on rest days require exclusion of an occupational cause for their asthma. If this is not possible with existing primary care resource locally, the case should be referred to a respiratory physician with an interest in occupational lung disease. Enclosing raw PEF data with the referral is invaluable.

MANAGEMENT

The general and pharmaceutical management of OA itself is similar to that for asthma not due to work, although overall case management is complex, as it involves not only the individual medical approach but also management of the workplace and any legislative aspects. This is beyond the scope of this chapter, but more detail is found in the standards of care for OA, linked to the British Thoracic Society website (www.brit-thoracic.org.uk).[2]

It is normal to advise removal of the worker with established OA from the harmful asthmagen exposure, or redeployment into a different workplace area with no exposure. This might be easy or difficult to achieve in practice.

Asthma aggravated in the workplace

Causes and common symptoms

Asthma symptoms (and control, therefore) might be worsened in the workplace by a variety of types of physical stimuli. For example, work involving greater levels of exercise than on rest days might aggravate asthma, particularly if the worker already has exercise-induced symptoms. Similarly, changes in temperature and humidity of the workplace (for example cold-room work, outdoor work) might worsen symptoms. Work with a variety of inhaled agents (irritant chemicals, dusts, aerosols) might also worsen asthma symptoms by a (presumably) variety of mechanisms.

What distinguishes asthma aggravated in the workplace from OA due to sensitisation is largely the rapid improvement seen in asthma symptoms following cessation of exposure in the workplace. Similarly, work-aggravated asthma does not tend to deteriorate with time even with repeated workplace exposure.

In practice, however, the distinction might be difficult (or occasionally impossible to be certain). Any doubt in relation to this difference would be a good reason to consider referral to a centre used to dealing with occupational lung diseases.

Initial investigations

These would be identical to those requested or started for workers with potential OA, as the distinction is normally based on interpreting objective measures, rather than relying on occupational and medical history alone.

Management

OA should be excluded, and then the workplace should be asked if adaptations could be made to reduce the triggering of asthma symptoms. Beta$_2$-agonists can be used as required prior to or during tasks known to be associated with worsening of asthma symptoms.

Acute irritant-Induced asthma

Causes

AIIA (formerly known as reactive airways dysfunction syndrome [RADS]) is generally considered to be an asthma-like state that occurs following (normally) a single large exposure to an irritant inhalation. Many different types of exposures are described. The symptoms of asthma normally begin within 24 hours following harmful exposure (for example a cloud of chlorine in a paper mill) and persist for at least 3 months.

Common symptoms

Symptoms are identical to those of normal asthma, although the onset is related very significantly to a single exposure event.

Initial investigations

The diagnosis is normally based on history, although other tests might be needed. In the first instance, if AIIA is suspected, a CXR and serial PEF monitoring should be performed. Airway reactivity measures are performed, but normally in a physiology laboratory.

Referral

As most workers with AIIA will require compensation advice, it is advisable to refer all such potential patients to a respiratory physician with an interest in occupational lung disease.

Management

There is very little evidence base to help here. It seems reasonable to treat with standard asthma medication during the period of symptoms (and probably for 3 years at least). The natural history of this condition is also not well understood, although some patients improve over time.

Key points: occupational asthma

▶ Always ask about job and job tasks in patients with persistent nasal symptoms.
▶ All healthcare workers should ask patients with airways disease about their current and previous work.
▶ All such patients should be asked about the nature of the agents with which they work. Patients should be allowed to describe these agents and their workplace conditions in their own words.
▶ All patients with respiratory symptoms who currently work should be asked about the work relationship of their symptoms (if any), in a neutral tone.
▶ A suggested wording for these questions is as follows: 'Is your (wheeze/chest tightness/shortness of breath/nasal irritation) the same, better or worse on your rest days/holidays?'
▶ The outlook for OA is better if workers are removed earlier from

exposure. All steps in the patient's journey contribute to potential delay.

▶ Make early referrals to a specialist with an interest in OA if such a diagnosis is suspected.

▶ All workers currently exposed to agents that can cause asthma and have work-related respiratory symptoms should undergo serial PEF measures. This can be initiated in primary care or in the occupational health setting, in addition to secondary care.

▶ Local expertise is likely to influence the local decision to investigate.

▶ A diagnosis of OA should never be based on history alone, and all reasonable attempts must be made to carry out objective tests.

▶ The pharmacological treatment of asthma is identical to that of non-OA. All physicians treating cases should not underestimate their power to prevent further cases by appropriate communication with legislators and workplaces, and by involvement in local education programmes.

▶ The index case of OA should not have further harmful exposure to the likely causative agent or process, and should prompt a full assessment of potential workplace exposures.

Source: adapted from Fishwick *et al.*[2]

Chronic obstructive pulmonary disease

Causes

COPD is a highly prevalent condition, and is dealt with in Chapter 8. This section deals with the interaction between COPD and the workplace.

Whilst the majority of COPD is caused by cigarette smoking, it is vital to remember that this condition has other causes and risk factors, including genetics and occupational exposures. In fact, there are many studies supporting the fact that on average 10–15 per cent of harm seen in this condition relates to harmful exposure to workplace vapours, dusts, gases and fumes (VDGF).

This is a difficult concept. Clearly, one in eight cases of COPD are not caused wholly by such exposures. Alternatively, workplace exposures to VDGF should be best thought of as causing additional respiratory damage, causing some workers to develop COPD, who had they 'just' smoked might not have developed this condition. In cases where occupational exposures have been very significant (or the individual worker very susceptible) they might be the predominant cause of COPD. Box 10.2 shows certain agents that are suspected of causing this occupational COPD 'effect'.

```
┌─────────────────────────────────────────────────────────────────┐
│ Box 10.2 ○  Specific agents suspected of causing occupational COPD │
├─────────────────────────────────────────────────────────────────┤
│  ▶ Coal dust.                                                     │
│  ▶ Silica dust.                                                   │
│  ▶ Cadmium.                                                       │
│  ▶ Grain.                                                         │
│  ▶ Cotton.                                                        │
│  ▶ Welding fumes.                                                 │
└─────────────────────────────────────────────────────────────────┘
```

Common symptoms

The symptoms of occupational COPD are no different from those of non-occupational COPD, and might well start many years after active work has stopped, due to the long latent period associated with its development. Chronic bronchitis, without evidence of airways obstruction, is also potentially linked to harmful workplace exposures, and the mechanism of sputum increase is likely to be similar to that caused by exposure to cigarette smoke.

Initial investigations

Investigations should be performed as per those for suspected COPD more generally. These would initially include (as a bare minimum) spirometry (FEV_1 and FVC) and a CXR. Further clues to the origin of disease might come from evidence of dust retention on CXR (pneumoconiosis) or of previous asbestos exposure. Routine pulmonary physiology will not help differentiate occupational from non-occupational causes. COPD in younger patients would suggest possible assessment of alpha 1 antitrypsin levels (AAT), and there is some evidence that VDGF workplace exposure and AAT deficiency interact to cause COPD in certain workers.

Referral

There are two main indications for referral for further assessment by a specialist:

▷ when occupational exposures are suspected as a significant cause of airways disease (and particularly if compensation issues are being discussed)

▷ when workers with COPD (or early airways disease) are working with VDGF. In this context, annual observation of FEV_1 would seem best practice. Whilst these measures might be taken by workplace-based practitioners as part of a health surveillance programme, this might not be the case. Workers with rapid loss of FEV_1 year on year (particularly if they smoke and are exposed to VDGF) are at higher risk of COPD.

Management

The general management of COPD is similar irrespective of the main cause in a given patient. Always ask a worker with chronic bronchitis if he or she is currently exposed in the workplace to VDGF, and never underestimate your ability as a healthcare professional to be able to influence this process. Local employers will respond to communications relating to the health of their workers, and this might have beneficial effects not only for the index case but also for all other workers harmfully exposed at the same workplace.

Key points: occupational COPD

▶ 10–15 per cent of the population burden of COPD relates to harmful occupational exposures to VDGF.
▶ Always ask a worker with chronic bronchitis if he or she is currently exposed in the workplace to VDGF.
▶ The harmful effects of occupation are most commonly seen in smokers, and probably interact to cause more lung damage.
▶ Identifying dusty workplaces and reducing the worker's exposure might lead to less rapid decline in FEV_1, even if the worker continues to smoke.
▶ Annual measures of FEV_1 might be difficult to interpret from the occupational point of view.
▶ 'Think COPD, think work!'

Extrinsic allergic alveolitis

Extrinsic allergic alveolitis (EAA) (also referred to as hypersensitivity pneumonitis) is a lung condition caused by an immunological reaction to an inhaled antigen, and separate from asthma. The immunology is more complex, but involves both lymphocytes and immune complex formation.

Causes

There are many occupational causes of EAA described. Table 10.1 lists some of the commonest occupational causes. Currently, the UK (as well as other countries) is experiencing outbreaks of EAA specifically related to metalworking fluid exposure. The exact cause of EAA in this group is not known, but is likely to relate to a contaminant. Metalworking fluids are used widely in industry, particularly where metals are being subjected to a grinding process to produce an end product (e.g. car manufacturing industry). Be especially vigilant, therefore, if patients working in such industries present with unexplained respiratory problems.

Table 10.1 ○ *Some causes of occupational EAA*

Farmer's lung	Mouldy hay
Air conditioner lung	Humidifier water
Metalworking fluid alveolitis	Contaminated metalworking fluid
Mushroom worker's lung	Mouldy mushroom compost
Malt worker's lung	Mouldy malt

Common symptoms

EAA typically occurs in acute, sub-acute and chronic forms. Symptoms of allergic alveolitis include chest tightness, shortness of breath, wheeze, rigors and sweats, muscles aches and malaise, flu-like symptoms and weight loss (with chronic disease). These symptoms might occur at work, or might be delayed for a few hours, and even start in the evening of workdays.

Initial investigations

A full set of blood investigations including C-reactive protein (CRP) and a CXR would be regarded as the minimum.

Referral

All suspected EAA should be referred to a respiratory physician with an interest in occupational lung disease.

Management

The management of this condition includes early removal from the workplace. Oral steroid treatment can be given to quicken improvement in the inflammatory process.

Pneumoconioses

Pneumoconiosis is a general term (although often inappropriately only applied to coal workers) to describe dust-related diseases. Broadly, dusts capable of causing a pneumoconiosis are divided into those that can cause significant fibrosis (fibrogenic) and those that do not generally cause fibrosis (non-fibrogenic).

Symptoms of cough and breathlessness might be a sign of significant fibrotic pneumoconiosis, even starting many years after last industrial exposure to dusts. A CXR is essential to diagnose (or suspect) pneumoconiosis. If the CXR shows evidence of small opacities, or more complex fibrosis, a full occupational history is likely to help decide the potential cause of the CXR abnormality.

Referral for further assessment and for assessment of pulmonary physiology is warranted for those with significant fibrosis. If practising in an area where coal mining, for example, was a common occupation, background changes of simple coal worker's pneumoconiosis might be very common. In this context, it seems reasonable to document CXR change only, if no other concerning features are present.

Table 10.2 lists common inhaled causes of both fibrogenic and non-fibrogenic pneumoconiosis.

Asbestos-related problems

Pleural plaques

Pleural plaques are commonly seen on CXR as an incidental finding in populations with previous asbestos exposure, typical in many industrial environments. They are only easily seen on CXR when they become calcified, and might develop over many years following cessation of asbestos exposure. They are collagenous hardenings of the parietal pleura, presumably caused by direct irritation of the pleural surface by asbestos fibres that reach this site. They are thought to be of no consequence, although act as a reliable marker of previous asbestos exposure.

The presence of pleural plaques in the absence of any other concerning feature would not normally require referral for further assessment. However, many patients with pleural plaque will have other respiratory problems and might have abnormal lung function. Additionally, compensation issues might be relevant. Consequently, referral for an opinion in relation to excluding more serious asbestos-related problems is justified in many circumstances.

Table 10.2 ○ *Common causes of pneumoconiosis*

Fibrogenic

Coal	Coal worker's pneumoconiosis
Silica	Silicosis
Asbestos	Asbestosis
Beryllium	Berylliosis

Non-fibrogenic

Iron	Siderosis
Tin	Stannosis
Barium	Baritosis

Pleural thickening and benign pleural effusions

Pleural thickening and effusions are a separate consequence of previous asbestos exposure and can present/develop many years after asbestos exposure. Radiology is not helpful at excluding an underlying neoplasm (lung cancer or mesothelioma) and as such all patients must be referred urgently for further assessment. Regional referral patterns vary, although it is likely that these referrals will be made urgently through the lung cancer referral pathways.

Asbestosis

Asbestosis is the term used to describe pulmonary fibrosis due to asbestos exposure. Practically, it behaves in a very similar way to pulmonary fibrosis not due to asbestos (termed cryptogenic fibrosing alveolitis), although it might be slower in its progression. All patients with significant fibrotic lung disease require referral for further assessment.

The treatment of asbestosis is difficult, although some patients might respond to oral steroid treatment.

CURRENT ASBESTOS EXPOSURE

Certain workers continue to be potentially exposed to asbestos at work. Although the use of new asbestos is not now possible, asbestos is still present in existing buildings. It is possible therefore that patients will present to you in primary care worried about recently identified asbestos exposure, normally as part of occupational exposure.

There are no easy rules to apply to such patients, as each case must be dealt with individually. Nevertheless, the risk to health of a single transient exposure to asbestos is generally regarded as low over a lifetime, and would not normally warrant a CXR, unless there are unexplained symptoms or signs.

The Health and Safety Executive (HSE) is actively interested in the area of asbestos exposure in workers and currently runs a campaign designed to reduce this, called 'Asbestos Kills: Protect Yourselves'.

This campaign essentially emphasises the future health risks of current asbestos exposure, the need to protect oneself, and not to disturb asbestos in buildings if this is possible. The associated literature offers a variety of practical advice for current workers at risk. The campaign focuses on electricians, plumbers, heating and ventilation engineers, joiners and general maintenance and building workers.

Further information can be sourced from HSE directly or on the appropriate website, the address of which is given at the end of this chapter.

Malignancy

Malignant mesothelioma

Malignant mesothelioma is a very unpleasant tumour of the pleura almost exclusively related to previous occupational or environmental asbestos exposure. There is also a rare peritoneal version of this tumour, again associated with asbestos exposure. Small numbers of these tumours might arise in patients without any previously likely or confirmed history of such exposure.

Presentation is typically a combination of shortness of breath and unilateral chest pain, often accompanied in the later stages with weight loss and anorexia. Physical signs are similar to those for a pleural effusion and the diagnosis is normally suggested at least from the findings on a CXR.

Lung cancer

Similar principles for lung cancer apply to COPD. Whilst the majority of lung cancer is attributable in population terms to cigarette smoking, various carcinogens met in the workplace increase the risk of lung cancer in certain workers. In population terms, 5–15 per cent of the total burden of lung cancer can be attributed to current and previous harmful workplace exposures. Whilst beyond the overall scope of this article, this message clearly has a preventive point. Reducing exposures to workplace carcinogens will reduce in time the numbers of new incident cases of lung cancer.

Box 10.3 lists the agents either known to cause lung cancer, or are suspected of doing so.

Box 10.3 ○ *Lung cancer at work – known or suspected agents*

▶ Inorganic arsenicals, nickel (during stainless steel and non-ferrous alloy manufacturing).
▶ Asbestos.
▶ Tin.
▶ Bischloromethyl ether.
▶ Zinc.
▶ Calcium or strontium chromate.
▶ Crystalline silica, radon, environmental tobacco smoke, mustard gas.
▶ Hematite, coke, soot, sulphuric acid mist, cadmium, particular dioxins, beryllium.

Other

Sick-building syndrome

Sick-building syndrome refers to a constellation of mucous membrane and respiratory symptoms that appear more frequent in workers occupying modern buildings in comparison with more historic, naturally ventilated buildings. Many other symptoms have also been reported to be commoner in office workers in modern buildings. Suspecting this in primary care might be difficult, and specialist referral in this context should probably be based around exclusion or confirmation of a particular diagnosis (e.g. asthma, rhinitis, conjunctivitis, bronchitis, COPD, etc. . . .).

The upper airway

Very little is known about the upper airway and occupational exposures, excluding clear diseases already discussed such as nasopharyngeal carcinoma in wood- or other workers. The upper airway is likely to be vulnerable (just like the lower respiratory tract) to the effects of irritant exposures in the workplace, and a condition known as reactive upper-airways disease is described. Practically, any worker complaining of work-related upper-airway irritation requires assessment, just like his or her non-occupational counterparts, to exclude more serious underlying diagnoses, prior to the workplace issues themselves being addressed.

Emerging conditions of interest

Recent novel diseases have been described, and it is essential to remain vigilant for any possible causes of lung disease in the workplace. Popcorn worker's lung is a type of respiratory disease probably due to exposure to diacetyl, which is used as a flavouring for popcorn.

Flock worker's lung is also described in workers cutting textile fibres (normally nylon) in a process for seating manufacture.

Compensation

Compensation for occupational lung diseases is a complex area, and patients with a potential claim need sensible, realistic advice. The law changes relatively often in relation to these issues, although good advice can be obtained from the Department for Work and Pensions (DWP) website (www.dwp.gov. uk), from trade unions, from personal injury lawyers with a specific interest in respiratory problems and from respiratory physicians with an interest in this area.

There might also be issues of limitation in cases of occupational lung disease. For example, in England, civil law might limit the progression of cases against those who negligently exposed workers to harmful workplace agents if the worker has known of his or her condition, and its relationship potentially to work for more than 3 years.

The message is simple: if you suspect occupational lung disease, refer to a centre that can give appropriate compensation advice (the patient should also consider asking the help of a personal injury lawyer). Also, advise the patient yourself that they *might* have a right to certain forms of compensation should a diagnosis of occupational lung disease be established, and document this advice in the case notes.

Workability

Whilst not strictly within the remit of this article, the workforce is ageing in tandem with the major population demographic change. These changes potentially have relevance for the workplace, as employers may have to deal both with adaptations required to employ older workers, and also to allow workers with chronic respiratory disease to carry on working. For example, those with milder COPD might wish to work for longer, and workplaces will have to consider how best to achieve this.

Primary care can play an important role in job retention for those with established respiratory disease, not least by good communication between yourselves, the workplace and occupational health professionals.

Communication

Good communication between relevant parties (e.g. primary care, secondary care, occupational health professionals, workplace managers, personnel, etc.) is key to improving the outcome in most cases of currently working patients with potential occupational lung disease. Whilst communicating (or copying correspondence) to as many interested parties as possible is the ideal, this should be done with the patient's consent.

Medical certification and reporting of cases

Medical certification for absence from work is no different for those with and without illness possibly caused or aggravated by the work environment. However, if a work connection is made in the written Form Med 3, there is then a legal requirement for the employer to act, including reporting the case to the HSE (see below). Consultation with patients suspected of (and indeed confirmed as having) occupational lung disease therefore affords an opportunity to communicate with the relevant workplace. The longer patients remain off work with a work-related illness, the less likely it is that they will return to work.

As part of a national reporting scheme, cases of occupational lung disease in England and Wales might be reported either by a volunteer occupational physician responsible for a worksite (Occupational Physicians Reporting Activity [OPRA] scheme), or by a secondary care-based respiratory physician (SWORD scheme). The scheme is now extending to primary care in certain areas. More information is available on the relevant website (shown at the end of this chapter).

Dealing with employers and changing the work environment

Employers have an obligation under Health and Safety law (under the Reporting of Injuries, Diseases and Dangerous Occurrences Regulations 1995 [RIDDOR] scheme) to report certain cases of work-related ill health such as occupational lung disorders to the HSE provided there is a written diagnosis from a medical practitioner, e.g. a Form Med 3. It is advisable to gain patient consent before divulging such information to a third party. Written diagnosis of this kind places a duty on the employer to take remedial action and, if reported, an HSE inspection could follow.

Occupational lung disease referral

Local secondary care-based centres might have specific occupational lung disease expertise, and the requirement for a specialist centre will depend on the nature of the case being referred and the specific investigation requirement. For example, the ability to perform specific inhalation challenge for OA is restricted to certain centres.

If local pathways of referral are not available, the Group of Occupational Respiratory Disease Specialists (GORDS) (secondary care-based respiratory physicians with an active clinical and research interest in OA and other occupational lung diseases) might be able to help further. Contact details are found at: www.hsl.gov.uk/cwh/gords.htm.

Further educational opportunity

BMJ e-learning currently offers a web-based OA e-learning package specifically designed for primary care,[3] and based around recent BOHRF guidance and the recent standards of care.[2]

Further self-assessment

Revisit your answers to the initial self-assessment. Would you amend any of them based on your learning?

When seeing a patient with history suggestive of asthma, list the occupations that would concern you that there might be an occupational cause.

A 70-year-old man has presented to your practice with unilateral chest pain and weight loss. He worked for many years in the power stations. Which initial investigations would you perform, and what single most likely diagnosis would you suggest (answer at end)?

Further resources

British Lung Foundation • **www.lunguk.org**.

British Occupational Health Research Foundation • **www.bohrf.org.uk**.

British Thoracic Society and Scottish Intercollegiate Guidelines Network. *British Guideline on the Management of Asthma: a national clinical guideline* London and Edinburgh: BTS and SIGN, 2008 • **www.brit-thoracic.org.uk/Portals/0/Clinical%20Information/ Asthma/Guidelines/asthma_final2008.pdf**.

Department for Work and Pensions, the Department of Health and the Health and Safety Executive. *Health, Work and Well-being: caring for our future. A strategy for the health and well-being of working age people* London: DWP, DH and HSE, 2005 • **www.dwp.gov.uk/publications/ dwp/2005/health_and_wellbeing.pdf**.

The Health and Occupation Reporting Network • **www.medicine. manchester.ac.uk/coeh/thor**.

Health and Safety Executive • **www.hse.gov.uk**.
  ▷ Health and Safety Executive Books [priced and free publications], PO Box 1999, Sudbury, Suffolk, CO10 2WA • **www.hsebooks.co.uk**.
  ▷ HSE infoline • **0845 345 0055**
  ▷ HSE, asbestos page • **www.hse.gov.uk/asbestos/index.htm**.
  ▷ HSE, asthma page • **www.hse.gov.uk/asthma/index.htm**.
  ▷ HSE, RIDDOR scheme • **www.hse.gov.uk/riddor**.
  ▷ HSE, Workplace Health Connect • **www.hse.gov.uk/workplacehealth/index.htm**.

207

References

1 • Nicholson PJ, Cullinan P, Taylor AJ, *et al*. Evidence based guidelines for the prevention, identification, and management of occupational asthma *Occupational and Environmental Medicine* 2005; **62(5)**: 290–9.

2 • Fishwick D, Barber CM, Bradshaw LM, *et al*. Standards of care for occupational asthma: British Thoracic Society Standards of Care Subcommittee Guidelines on Occupational Asthma *Thorax* 2008; **63(3)**: 240–50. Epub 2007 Sep 28.

3 • BMJ Learning. Occupational asthma: evidence based diagnosis and management [interactive case history], http://learning.bmj.com/learning/search-result. html?moduleId=6051298 [accessed January 2009].

Further self-assessment: answer

This is a typical history of malignant mesothelioma, or lung cancer with internal chest wall invasion. Other less likely diagnoses include pleural or pulmonary tuberculosis, empyema or benign pleural thickening.

Initial investigations should include blood testing (including erythrocyte sedimentation rate and CRP) and a CXR. Malignant mesothelioma is almost always associated with pleural thickening and effusion seen on radiology, and should prompt an immediate urgent referral for exclusion of malignancy.

Occupational exposure to asbestos is normally seen in those with malignant mesothelioma, and power station work would have normally been associated historically with some asbestos exposure (for example pipe laggers using asbestos to lag pipes for thermal insulation).

Respiratory infections and other common lung diseases

11

Simon Gregory

Introduction

Respiratory infections are the commonest infective cause of general practice consultations, accounting for 25 per cent of a GP's workload and 30 per cent of all hospital admissions. Such infections range from minor self-limiting upper respiratory tract infections (URTIs) to the more serious community-acquired pneumonia (CAP) and tuberculosis (TB). In children most respiratory infections affect the upper respiratory tract. Such infections decline with age whereas lower respiratory tract infections (LRTIs) increase with age. It is vital that GPs are competent to diagnose and treat respiratory infections, and to know when and when not to prescribe.

Chapter aims

This chapter aims to cover the breadth of respiratory infections, and some other key lung disorders that are not covered in other chapters, to sufficient depth to inform your practice as a GP.

Learning outcomes

After reading this chapter you will have refreshed your knowledge of:

▷ URTIs
▷ LRTIs
▷ bronchitis and CAP
▷ TB
▷ fungal respiratory disease
▷ bronchiectasis
▷ sarcoidosis.

Initial self-assessment

Before reading this chapter we suggest that you consider the following questions. After reading the chapter you might wish to revisit your answers.

1 ▷ What are the clinical features of a patient presenting with a sore throat that would make you consider prescribing an antibiotic?

2 ▷ How would you differentiate clinically between bronchitis and CAP?

3 ▷ You are called to visit an 80-year-old woman who lives alone in her own home. She has CAP. Which factors would encourage you to arrange hospital referral?

4 ▷ What health promotion measures might a practice employ to reduce the incidence of respiratory tract infections in the population it serves?

Upper respiratory tract infections

URTIs are defined as those that occur above the vocal cords. These are common all year round but especially in the winter months. The majority of URTIs are caused by picornaviruses, that is rhinovirus (40 per cent) and coxsackie viruses. Other causative viruses include adenoviruses, coronaviruses (15 per cent), echoviruses, influenza, para-influenza and respiratory syncytial virus (RSV).

The commonest URTI is the 'common cold'. This is transmitted by droplet spread and hand or facial contact. It presents with coryza (runny nose), a cough and a sore throat. The illness is self-limiting unless complicated by a supra-added infection. Therefore management is conservative. That is, patients should be helped to manage their symptoms but do not require active medical intervention. Pharmacists are ideally suited to provide such assistance.

Sore throat

Most cases of sore throat are also viral; a minority are bacterial, of which group A beta-haemolytic streptococci are the commonest bacterial pathogen (hence the US vernacular 'strep throat'). Patients typically present with a sore throat, anorexia, headache, malaise and otalgia. There may be tonsillitis or pharyngitis but exudate on the tonsil does not confirm the presence of bacteria, despite historically this perhaps being a trigger for the prescription of antibiotics. The Centor criteria were developed to help indicate which throat infections might be due to group A streptococci.[1] These four criteria can act as an aid to diagnosis (Box 11.1), but even these only give a poor indication of the likelihood of bacterial causation. If there is massive exudate, typically combined with significant generalised lymphadenopathy, then infectious mononucleosis should be included in the differential diagnosis. If considering the use of antibiotics in the UK it is worth remembering that the number needed to treat (NNT) is 7. It is important if you choose to work abroad that this situation might not apply. Management of acute RTIs in the past concentrated on advising prompt antibiotic treatment of presumptive bacterial infections. This advice was appropriate in an era of high rates of serious suppurative and non-suppurative complications (such as rheumatic fever), up to and including the immediate post-war period. However, in modern developed countries, rates of major complications are now low.[2] If you choose to work abroad this change might not apply.

Box 11.1 ○ *Centor criteria*

According to the number of criteria present:
▶ absence of cough
▶ fever
▶ tender anterior cervical nodes
▶ purulent pharynx (exudate).

Number of criteria present = % chance of a streptococcal infection
0 = 25%, 1 = 38%, 2 = 40%, 3 = 53%, 4 = 67%

Rhinosinusitis

Historically this was referred to as sinusitis as it is typified by an inflammation of the mucous membranes of the para-nasal sinuses but the term rhinosinusitis is more accurate as the nasal mucosa is also inflamed. This inflammation might be due to local irritation, infection or allergy. It typically presents with nasal congestion and/or a runny nose, sinus pain and fever. It might be accompanied by tenderness over the sinuses. In considering the management, predisposing factors include atopy, occupational exposure, nasal polyps or a deviated nasal septum and smoking.

Chronic rhinosinusitis is normally irritant or allergic in nature and is therefore normally treated with antihistamines or inhaled nasal corticosteroids, but care should be taken not to neglect addressing the underlying causation, including the possibility of there being an underlying fungal infection.

Acute sinusitis is normally of infective origin but it is important to note that more than 60 per cent of cases resolve without antibiotic treatment. A common theme in the treatment of respiratory infections is the mismatch between the patient's expectation of antibiotics and the doctor's perception of that expectation. Doctors typically overestimate the patient's desire for such drugs. It is important to elicit the patient's health beliefs, his or her concerns and his or her desired outcome of the consultation. Antibiotics should be reserved for those patients with severe symptoms or signs, who are systemically unwell or those who are worsening rather than improving. Symptom resolution might be slow however and can take 2 or more weeks.

Epiglottitis

Type B *Haemophilus influenzae* can cause a life-threatening infection of the supra-glottic larynx. This is rare over the age of 5 years old and is much rarer since the introduction of the Hib vaccination programme. It is included here as it is vital not to miss it, and paradoxically with it becoming less common it might come to mind less readily. The child is extremely ill with a high fever and airflow obstruction. The throat must not be examined until there are facilities to maintain the airway.

Management strategies

Whether to prescribe an antibiotic or not for a respiratory tract infection is but one component of the management of these conditions. The patient or carer should be involved in the determination of the management plan. The NICE clinical guideline on respiratory tract infections offers excellent advice on such management,[2] including:

- ▶ clinical assessment
- ▶ determining and addressing ideas, concerns and expectations
- ▶ appropriate antibiotic use strategies, such as
  - ▷ no prescription
  - ▷ provision of a delayed prescription
  - ▷ immediate antibiotic prescription issue and appropriate clinical review.

Lower respiratory tract infections

These typically include acute bronchitis and pneumonia. Community-acquired LRTIs are generally caused by viral infections, but other causative agents include bacteria and atypical pathogens. The incidence is reported as being 44 cases per 1000 population per annum.[3] The incidence is 2–4 times higher in people aged 60 and over than in those aged under 50. Placebo-controlled trials have shown little or no benefit in treating uncomplicated LRTIs with antibiotics in previously well patients.[4] This should not be applied to CAP (see p. 214). In contrast with URTIs in which the evidence of patient desire for an antibiotic is weaker when presenting with acute lower respiratory symptoms most patients believe that their symptoms are caused by an infection and that antibiotics will help. Three-quarters of previously well adult patients with such symptoms receive antibiotics even though their GPs believe they are only indicated in a fifth of cases. Patients who do not receive an antibiotic are more likely to be dissatisfied, and dissatisfied patients re-consult twice as frequently.[5] The authors of this study suggest that terms such as bronchitis and chest infection as explanations to the patient might be unhelpful and that patient education is vital. As patient choice and satisfaction surveys are now a major component of government thinking, yet antibiotic over-prescribing is a major concern, we will need to consider how we communicate and how we educate patients presenting with these symptoms.

Acute bronchitis

Acute bronchitis refers to inflammation of the bronchi. The typical symptom complex is of a productive cough (yellow/green sputum), pyrexia, fatigue, dyspnoea on exertion and possibly wheezing. It occurs more frequently in the winter months. Predisposing factors include smoking, pollution, lower socioeconomic groups and overcrowded housing. The most common causative agents are viral but, in common with other LRTIs, patients typically consider infection to be synonymous with the need for antibiotics and they are typically prescribed. Viruses involved include RSV, influenza, para-influenza, rhinoviruses and picornaviruses (rhinovirus). Bacterial causes include *Haemophilus influenzae*, *Streptococcus pneumoniae* and *Moraxella catarrhalis*. Physical signs include pyrexia, basal crackles and polyphonic expiratory wheezing. If antibiotics are indicated the guidelines extant at the time and location should be followed but in general amoxicillin or erythromycin are those most commonly employed.

Pneumonia

Pneumonia is an inflammation of the substance of the lungs. Typically this is infection involving the alveoli with resulting consolidation. Thus consolidation differentiates pneumonia from bronchitis. Pneumonias are commonly classified according to the probable origin of the infection:

▷ CAP
▷ hospital acquired (nosocomial)
▷ immunosuppressed patients
▷ chemical (e.g. aspiration pneumonia)
▷ radiotherapy
▷ allergic.

In this chapter we focus on CAP as it is this that we commonly meet as general practitioners (GPs). TB can also be considered as a form of CAP but is considered separately as its patho-physiology, presentation and treatment are quite different.

Community-acquired pneumonia

CAP (in the community) is defined as having the following features:[6]

▷ symptoms of an acute lower respiratory tract illness (cough and at least one other lower respiratory tract symptom)
▷ new focal chest signs on examination
▷ at least one systemic feature (either a symptom complex of sweating, fevers, shivers, aches and pains and/or temperature of 38°C or more)
▷ no other explanation for the illness . . . .

The annual incidence in the community is 5–11 per 1000 adult population; this counts for between 5 and 12 per cent of LRTIs managed by GPs. The incidence is higher in the young and the elderly. Only 1 in 6 patients typically require admission to hospital and the mortality rate is about 5 per cent.

In adults CAP is typically caused by *Streptococcus pneumoniae* (19.3 per cent), *Mycoplasma pneumoniae* (11.1 per cent), *Chlamydia pneumoniae* (8 per cent), and *Haemophilus influenzae* (3.3 per cent). In 49.8 per cent of cases no pathogen is identified.[7] In children the cause is more typically viral.

The clinical features of CAP are shown in Table 11.1. The illness typically begins with fever and rigors, and sometimes pleuritic chest pain. However, it can present with a cough of several day's duration. In the elderly there might be no respiratory symptoms but abnormal signs found on chest examination.[8]

Table 11.1 ○ *Clinical features of community-acquired pneumonia*[6]

Respiratory symptoms	%	Non-respiratory symptoms	%	Signs	%
Cough	90	Vomiting	20	Fever	80+
Sputum	70	Confusion	15	Tachypnoea	80+
Dyspnoea	70	Diarrhoea	15	Tachycardia	80+
Chest pain	65	Rash	5	Abnormal chest signs	80+
Upper respiratory symptoms	33	Abdominal pain	5	Hypotension	20
Haemoptysis	15			Confusion	15
				Herpes labialis	10

The British Thoracic Society CAP guidelines[6] list specific clinical features that might be associated with specific pathogens (Table 11.2). These should be used to encourage lateral thought to possible causes and aid management, but should not be taken too literally as there is a considerable body of litera-ture which suggests that there is no strong correlation.[9]

Historically some pneumonias were described as being atypical. This was said to include the following infective agents: *Mycoplasma pneumoniae, Chlamydia pneumoniae, Chlamydia psittaci, Coxiella burnetii* and *Leigionella* spp. However, later evidence suggests that these cannot be clearly differentiated based on symptoms or signs and that there is considerable overlap between typical and atypical pneumonias. The term 'atypical' should be discarded as unhelpful, and *Legionella* is of sufficient import that it should be considered separately (see p. 217).

Investigations are not normally required in the community unless the patient is seriously ill. In such cases hospital admission might be indicated. Sputum examination and a chest X-ray might be of use if a patient does not respond to treatment. A leucocytosis and a raised C-reactive protein might aid differential diagnosis. Liver function tests might aid consideration of multi-system disease and serum urea helps assist severity but is no longer available in the community in many areas. Pulse oximetry is now reason-ably priced and readily available, and therefore can form a useful adjunct to

Table 11.2 ○ *Specific clinical features of respiratory pathogens*[4]

Streptococcus pneumoniae	▶ Increasing age ▶ Co-morbidity ▶ Acute onset ▶ High fever ▶ Pleuritic chest pain
Bacteraemic *Streptococcus pneumoniae*	▶ Female gender ▶ Alcohol excess ▶ Diabetes mellitus ▶ COPD ▶ Dry cough
Legionella pneumophila	▶ Younger patients ▶ Smoker ▶ Absence of co-morbidity ▶ Diarrhoea ▶ Neurological symptoms ▶ More severe infection with evidence of multi-system involvement, e.g. abnormal liver function tests or raised creatine kinase
Mycoplasma pneumoniae	▶ Younger patients ▶ Prior antibiotics ▶ Less multi-system involvement
Chlamydia pneumoniae	▶ Longer duration of symptoms ▶ Headache
Coxiella burnetti	▶ Male gender ▶ Dry cough ▶ High fever

the assessment of severity. Hypoxaemia (SpO$_2$ of <92 per cent in patients who are normally at higher levels) is a concerning prognostic indicator that would normally suggest the need for assertive management, usually hospital admission.

The severity of CAP can be assessed using the CURB-65 tool. Since this includes the measurement of serum urea it has been adapted to the CRB-65 tool for use in general practice (Figure 11.1). This is an aid to, not a substitute for, clinical judgement and patient preference.

The initial management and choice of antibiotic should be guided by the clinical assessment and in line with local guidelines and patterns of antibiotic resistance. For mild CAP amoxicillin or erythromycin still form the mainstay of treatment, though typically in higher doses and for longer periods than in bronchitis (amoxicillin 500 mg three times daily or erythromycin 500 mg four times daily for 7 days). In severely ill patients and those with

Figure 11.1 ○ *CRB-65 prognostic indicator for management of CAP*

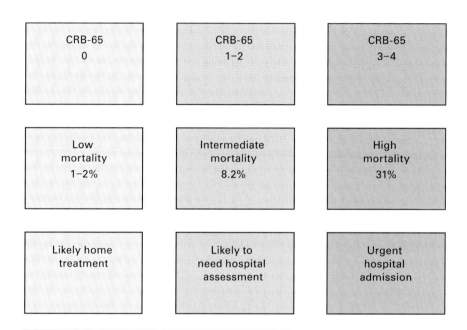

Prognostic features:
▸ increased **C**onfusion
▸ **R**espiratory rate >30/min
▸ **B**lood pressure (systolic <90 or diastolic <60 mmHg
▸ age ≥ **65** years

| CRB-65 0 | CRB-65 1–2 | CRB-65 3–4 |

| Low mortality 1–2% | Intermediate mortality 8.2% | High mortality 31% |

| Likely home treatment | Likely to need hospital assessment | Urgent hospital admission |

Source: adapted from the British Thoracic Society.[10]

co-morbidity longer courses might be needed. Sputum culture is indicated for those patients who do not respond to empirical treatment. Patients with suspected CAP should also be advised to rest and drink plenty of fluids, and should be advised against smoking.

Legionella pneumonia (Legionnaire's disease)

Legionella pneumophila was first identified in January 1977 following an outbreak of a severe variant of pneumonia at a convention of American Legionnaires in Philadelphia. It is a bacterium, which thrives in warm, still water environments (25–45°C). Air-conditioning systems typify such environments as they both support propagation and readily disseminate the *Legionella* sp. Whilst outbreaks gain media and public attention, single cases are themselves common. In the UK 40 per cent of patients have recently returned from travelling overseas. Whilst there might only be a mild flu-like illness (Pontiac fever) pneumonia can ensue. This is typically a more severe illness, and even with the correct treatment one that is slow to resolve. The features are shown in Table 11.2. This should be considered whenever patients are deteriorating or not responding to treatment, especially in younger patients and those who develop multi-system disease. Urgent admission is indicated and once admitted rapid *Legionella* urine antigen testing should be performed. *Legionella pneumonia* should not knowingly be managed in the community. Current treatments include quinolone or newer macrolide antibiotics and on some occasions rifampicin.

Prevention of pneumonia

Chronic lung disease is a major pre-determinant of pneumonia and therefore the most important controllable risk factor is tobacco smoking (see Chapter 3). Influenza vaccination is recommended for the elderly and those with diabetes mellitus and chronic lung, heart and kidney disease. Pneumococcal vaccination is also recommended for those at risk, especially older patients and those without a spleen.

Other important factors are legal restrictions and design improvements regarding building design and water-system design, and restrictions on the transport and import of exotic birds.

Pulmonary tuberculosis

TB is the second highest cause of death worldwide, causing 1.6 million deaths in 2005. It is estimated that 2 billion people are infected. TB is spread by airborne dissemination of droplets containing *Mycobacterium tuberculosis*. Once inhaled these deposit in the distal airways. The patho-physiology of the disease is not covered herein as it is not critical to the understanding or management of the disease in primary care and is well covered elsewhere.

Typical features include cough, sputum (muco-purulent), haemoptysis, fever, weight loss and malaise. There might also be apical crackles, anorexia, focal wheezing and chest wall pain. In some cases there are no symptoms. The presentations of TB are protean. It is known as the great mimic. Making the diagnosis depends on clinical suspicion including history, clinical and radiological investigation combined with tuberculin testing and microbiological investigations (isolation of the mycobacterium is essential to confirm diagnosis, to inform treatment particularly regarding sensitivities, to assess infectivity and to prove links between cases). At least three sputum samples are required, at least one of which should be an early morning sample. A normal chest X-ray almost excludes pulmonary TB. Inactivity of disease cannot be determined from radiographs.

TB is particularly common in minority ethnic populations, especially those from Asia and sub-Saharan Africa. There are therefore health-screening programmes for new entrants to the UK. Clinicians should consider new immigrants to be at greater risk for 5 years after entry.

Patients with respiratory symptoms or who are generally unwell must be investigated, and those with active disease must be treated. Contact tracing is essential. Public health departments in conjunction with departments of respiratory medicine conduct this. Contacts typically undergo tuberculin testing and chest radiography, and are retested after two months. There is also now a blood test for latent disease. If testing is positive then chemoprophylaxis is indicated.

TB is a notifiable disease: notification compulsory upon suspicion rather than confirmation. Furthermore, the Public Health (Control of Diseases) Act 1984 provides a legal basis for requiring compulsory examination of symptomatic patients, enforced hospitalisation of patients 'in an infectious state' and post-mortem examinations if required.

In the UK the standard recommended treatment regimen is 6 months of isoniazid and rifampicin plus pyrazinamide and ethambutol for the first 2 months.[11] GPs are not commonly involved in the prescription or administration of anti-tuberculous medication as a respiratory physician should prescribe it, but support of the GP can greatly aid adherence. Combination tablets and daily dosing regimes are the recommended first choice for treatment. Thrice-weekly directly observed treatment (DOT) should be considered for those patients with adverse factors, such as homeless people or those who are likely to have poor adherence. Other approaches to improve adherence with anti-tuberculous regimens are shown in Box 11.2. It is vital that an adherence risk assessment is conducted for all TB patients as poor adherence with so prolonged a programme and consequent drug resistance are a major personal and public health problem. Treatment failure is not uncommon.

> **Box 11.2** ○ *Interventions to improve adherence with anti-tuberculous therapy*
>
> ▶ Directly observed therapy.
> ▶ Clear explanation (health education counselling).
> ▶ Reminder letters (in appropriate languages).
> ▶ Patient-centred interview and health education booklet.
> ▶ Patient diary.
> ▶ TB health visitor domiciliary visits.
> ▶ Monitoring including random urine tests and medicine counting.
> ▶ Support with gaining benefits and help with prescription costs.
>
> *Source*: amended from Fang *et al.*[9]

Surgery is seldom required but might be indicated if there is localised drug-resistant disease, localised previous TB mycetoma or empyema.

Fungal respiratory disease

Fungi cause a variety of lung diseases. Causative agents include *Aspergillus, Pneumocystis jiroveci* (formerly *carinii*) and *Cryptococcus*. There are other mycoses, which are endemic to North America, but these are not covered herein.

Aspergillus spp. are ubiquitous environmental moulds that grow on organic matter and aerosolise.[12] These fungi cause a variety of clinical syndromes:

1 ▷ **allergy** • atopic allergy to fungal spores (IgE mediated). About 10 per cent of asthmatics are skin prick positive to *Aspergillus* and mould sensitivity has been associated with increased severity of asthma. High exposure results from working with mouldy vegetable matter such as compost heaps

2 ▷ *Aspergillus*-**driven asthma** • that is, allergy with IgE and IgG positive reaction. It is suggested that *Aspergillus* spores germinate within the airways triggering an enhanced asthmatic reaction. Management includes either inhaled or oral corticosteroids. There is little evidence of improvement with antifungal agents

3 ▷ **allergic bronchopulmonary aspergillosis** • this might be an extreme form of *Aspergillus*-driven asthma. In addition to a history of asthma and IgE and IgG there is proximal bronchiectasis. Patients typically have a recent deterioration of asthma with fever and malaise. There are recurrent episodes of mucous plugging; these plugs are often expectorated and are darker than usual mucous

plugs. There might also be eosinophilia and haemoptysis. Treatment consists of the management of severe asthma (see Chapter 4)
combined with prolonged courses of itraconazole with appropriate
liver function test monitoring

4 ▷ **aspergilloma** • this typically occurs as presumed colonisation
of a previously present cavity. They are often asymptomatic. Most
that are symptomatic present with haemoptysis

5 ▷ **invasive aspergillosis** • this is normally only found in the
immunocompromised patient. The hyphae of the *Aspergillus*
invade the tissues. Features typically include cough, chest pain,
fever, dyspnoea and haemoptysis. This is a specialist area and such
patients should be sent promptly to the physician managing the
underlying cause of their immunosuppression

6 ▷ **semi-invasive aspergillosis** • it is assumed that this is due to
lowered immunity but not true immunosuppression. Mycelial
balls are commonly found with progressive fibrosis but minimal
fungal invasion. In this situation steroids are not to be used as mild
immunosuppression is thought to be the underlying cause. Oral
antifungals are therefore indicated.

Pneumocystis carinii pneumonia (PCP) is still called this despite the name
change of the infective agent to *Pneumocystis jiroveci. P. jiroveci* is a widespread
environmental pathogen, which most people have encountered by the age
of 2. PCP is thought to result from new infection. It occurs in immunocompromised patients, especially those with HIV infection. Features include a
dry cough and exertional breathlessness with fever and tachypnoea, but
typically chest clinical examination is unremarkable. Management is by
specialist units. It usually includes high-dose co-trimoxazole.

Bronchiectasis

Bronchiectasis is irreversible destructive lung disease that is characterised
by abnormal dilatation of one or more bronchi with persistent inflammation. It should be suspected in any patient with recurrent LRTIs and sputum
production. The prevalence is unknown. Diagnosis was made on the basis of
radiographical evidence. This was likely to be an under-estimate. Thin-sec-
tion high-resolution CT (HRCT) scanning is now the investigation of choice.
This might diagnose more minor cases thus raising the apparent prevalence.
Perhaps a third of patients with COPD might have bronchiectasis were they
to have HRCT scans. Dilatation of bronchi, mucous gland hyperplasia and

ciliary hypoplasia create an environment in which bacteria proliferate. The process becomes self-perpetuating.

During exacerbations patients develop a productive cough with mucopurulent sputum that is associated with breathlessness and haemoptysis. Signs typically include coarse (low-pitched) inspiratory and expiratory crackles and wheezes. Whilst finger clubbing is recognised in bronchiectasis it is only found in the most severe cases.

Box 11.3 ○ *Causes of bronchiectasis*

▶ **Genetic** • cystic fibrosis, alpha 1-antitrypsin deficiency.
▶ **Mucociliary** • primary ciliary dyskinesia, Kartagener's syndrome, Young's syndrome.
▶ **Post-infective** • TB, measles, pertussis, severe pneumonia.
▶ **Immune deficiency** • immunoglobulin deficiency, HIV.
▶ **Other** • aspiration, tumour, toxic inhalation, coeliac disease.

Investigations of possible bronchiectasis include chest X-ray, HRCT scan, barium swallow, lung function tests, sputum microbiology and full-blood count (differential white-cell count).

Treatment depends upon the severity of the disease. Influenza and pneumococcal vaccination are vital. Inhaled bronchodilators can be used if there is demonstrable reversibility but inhaled corticosteroids seem to be of little benefit. Antibiotics should be reserved for when there are exacerbations including increased production of purulent sputum. As with COPD higher doses of antibiotics are required to achieve tissue penetration. In bronchiectasis there is typically a high pathogen load. Antimicrobial therapy should be tailored to the colonising organism. Whilst local guidelines and resistance patterns should be noted, typically amoxicillin 500 mg t.d.s. for 10–14 days is required. If pseudomonas is isolated then ciprofloxacin 750 mg b.d. p.o. for 2 weeks is normally required.

Surgery can be indicated but this is typically only the case if the bronchial damage is localised and there is no persistent underlying cause.

Pulmonary sarcoidosis

Sarcoidosis is a multi-system inflammatory disorder that is typified by the presence of non-caseating granulomata. It commonly involves the respiratory system but can actually affect any system. It typically occurs in young adults with a peak incidence in the third and fourth decades. It is more common in females than males and is more common in those of African and Caribbean descent and the Irish. It is also typically a more aggressive disease in black populations.

Pulmonary sarcoidosis can be asymptomatic with the typical bilateral hilar lymphadenopathy being found on a routine chest X-ray. Or the bilateral hilar lymphadenopathy might be found in patients presenting with erythema nodosum and anterior uveitis. Indeed if erythema nodosum is found in the 20 to 40 age group it might be considered to be sarcoidosis until proven otherwise, and similarly so with anterior uveitis. Patients might present with pulmonary symptoms, including cough and dyspnoea, and bilateral hilar lymphadenopathy then be found on chest X-ray. Fatigue, weight loss, peripheral lympadenopathy and fever might also be reported. Examination should be targeted at the above features, particularly for skin and eye lesions, lymphadenopathy and hepatosplenomegaly.

Respiratory physicians will typically perform a range of investigations including chest X-ray, Mantoux test (to exclude tuberculosis), serum angiotensin-converting enzyme (a surrogate marker of sarcoid inflammation), and lung function tests. They might also perform HRCT to assess if there are pulmonary infiltrates.

Extra-pulmonary disease might affect any system. Skin and eye involvement is the most common as has been mentioned above. Other features include the central nervous system (Bell's palsy, lymphocytic meningitis), liver/spleen (hepatosplenomegaly, portal hypertension), cardiovascular (cardiomyopathy), renal (nephrolithiasis, interstitial nephritis), musculoskeletal (polyarthritis, myositis), metabolic (hypercalcaemia). Sarcoidosis is therefore a complex disease and as such should be managed by appropriate specialists.

Most patients with pulmonary sarcoidosis do not require treatment. Commonly the pulmonary disease is simply monitored. If treatment is required then the mainstay of treatment is immunosuppression with corticosteroids. It is suggested that two therapeutic pitfalls might trap the unwary clinician: over-treatment and under-treatment.[13] Typically treatment starts with 40 mg daily for about 4 weeks but a maintenance dose of 5–15 mg might be required for 6–12 months. Care should be taken to remember the adverse effects of steroids. In particular gastric protection and osteoporosis prevention should be considered. If steroid treatment fails or the disease becomes life threatening other immunosuppressive treatments might be required.

The prognosis of pulmonary sarcoidosis is typically good. It usually remits within 2 years in more than two-thirds of patients with hilar lymphadenopathy alone. The disease is fatal in less than 3 per cent of UK cases, in those cases being due to respiratory failure or rarely from myocardial sarcoidosis or renal involvement. The prognosis is much worse in certain ethnic groups. In black patients in the USA it is as high as 10 per cent.

Further self-assessment

1 ▷ Revisit your answers to the initial self-assessment. Would you amend any of them based on your learning?
2 ▷ When seeing a patient with history suggestive of pneumonia, what would make you consider a diagnosis of:
   a • Legionnaire's disease?
   b • TB?
3 ▷ A 37-year-old man who has recently joined your practice list is already on treatment for pulmonary TB and under the care of the local TB team. What involvement would you expect to have? How would you assess medication adherence? How might you encourage accurate completion of the medication course?

Further resources

COMMUNITY-ACQUIRED PNEUMONIA

BTS Pneumonia Guidelines Committee. *BTS Guidelines for the Management of Community Acquired Pneumonia in Adults* London: BTS, 2004 • **www.brit-thoracic.org.uk/ClinicalInformation/Pneumonia/PneumoniaGuidelines/tabid/136/Default.aspx** • [accessed January 2009].

TUBERCULOSIS

National Institute for Health and Clinical Excellence. *Clinical Guideline 33, Tuberculosis* London: NICE, 2006 • **www.nice.org.uk/nicemedia/pdf/CG033niceguideline.pdf** • [accessed January 2009].

INFECTIONS

National Electronic Library of Infection • **www.neli.org.uk** • [accessed January 2009].

Further reading

Zambon M. Influenza, respiratory syncytial virus and SARS *Medicine* 2005; **33**: 130–4.

References

1 • Centor R M, Witherspoon J M, Dalton H P, *et al*. The diagnosis of strep throat in adults in the emergency room *Medical Decision Making* 1981; **1(3)**: 239–46.

2 • National Institute for Health and Clinical Excellence. *Clinical Guideline 69, Respiratory Tract Infections – antibiotic prescribing. Prescribing of antibiotics for self-limiting respiratory tract infections in adults and children in primary care* London: NICE, 2008.

3 • Macfarlane J T, Colville A, Gioun A, *et al*. Prospective study of aetiology and outcome of adult lower-respiratory-tract infections in the community *Lancet* 1993; **341**: 511–14.

4 • Orr P H, Scherer K, Macdonald A, *et al*. Randomised placebo controlled trials of antibiotics for acute bronchitis: a critical review of the literature *Family Practice* 1993; **36**: 507–12.

5 • Macfarlane J, Holmes W, Macfarlane R, *et al*. Influence of patients' expectations on antibiotic management of acute lower respiratory tract illness in general practice: questionnaire study *British Medical Journal* 1997; **315**: 1211–14.

6 • British Thoracic Society. Guidelines for the management of community acquired pneumonia in adults *Thorax* 2001; **56 (suppl. IV)**.

7 • Woodhead M. Community-acquired pneumonia in Europe: causative pathogens and resistance patterns *European Respiratory Journal* 2002; **20(suppl 36)**: 20s–27s.

8 • Wilkinson M, Woodhead M. *Pneumonia Medicine* 2004; **32**: 129–34.

9 • Fang G D, Fine M, Orloff J, *et al*. New and emerging etiologies for community acquired pneumonia with implications for therapy. A prospective multicenter study of 369 cases *Medicine* 1990; **69**: 307–16.

10 • BTS Pneumonia Guidelines Committee. *BTS Guidelines for the Management of Community Acquired Pneumonia in Adults* London: BTS, 2004, www.brit-thoracic.org.uk/ClinicalInformation/Pneumonia/PneumoniaGuidelines/tabid/136/Default.aspx [accessed January 2009].

11 • National Institute for Health and Clinical Excellence. *Clinical Guideline 33, Tuberculosis* London: NICE, 2006, www.nice.org.uk/nicemedia/pdf/CG033niceguideline.pdf [accessed January 2009].

12 • Barnes P D, Marr K A. Aspergillosis: spectrum of disease, diagnosis and treatment *Infectious Disease Clinics of North America* 2006; **20**: 545–61.

13 • Fitzgerald M X. Pulmonary sarcoidosis *Medicine* 2004; **32**: 148–52.

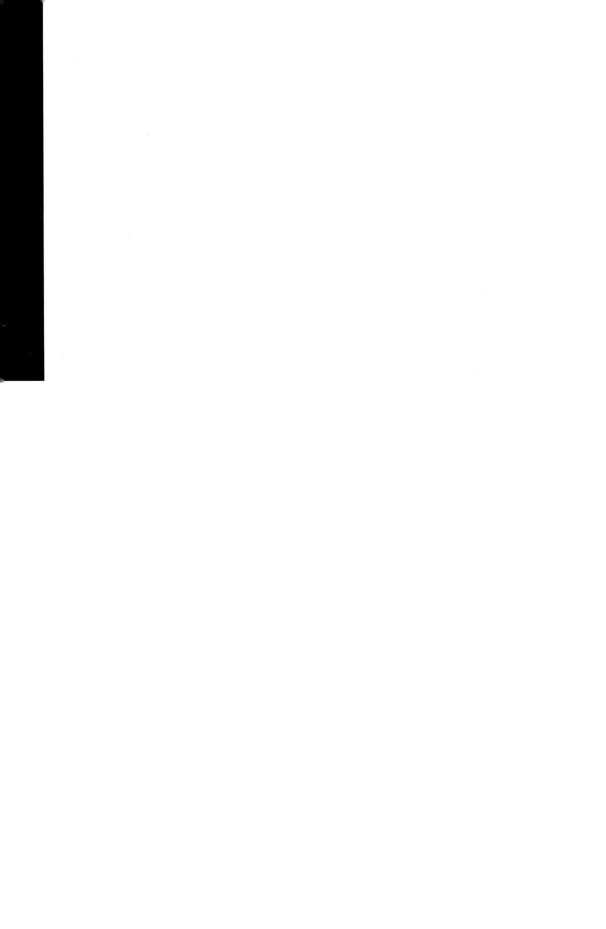

Oxygen therapy

12

Yvonne Henderson

Chapter aims

This chapter aims to enable you to understand the complex issues surrounding the use of oxygen therapy as part of the management of acute and chronic respiratory disease in primary care and community settings. It gives guidelines for patient assessment to ensure the appropriate prescription, delivery and monitoring of oxygen therapy, and describes current national guidelines.

Learning outcomes

At the end of this chapter you will be able to understand:

▷ the role of oxygen therapy in both acute and chronic disease management
▷ the process involved in assessing a patient's oxygen requirements and selecting a delivery device to ensure appropriate oxygen therapy is given
▷ the current national guidelines for oxygen prescription in primary care.

Initial self-assessment

Many doctors are used to prescribing short-term oxygen therapy in secondary care settings, but how prepared are you for prescribing oxygen as a GP?

For each of the following questions more than one answer might be correct. The answers are within this chapter.

Q1) Which of the following can lead to inaccurate pulse oximetry readings?

A ▷ Jaundice
B ▷ Pigmented skin
C ▷ Shivering
D ▷ Nail varnish
E ▷ Anaemia

Key ▶ **C, D**

Q2) For how many hours per day should long-term oxygen therapy be used?

  A ▷ 3

  B ▷ 6

  C ▷ 12

  D ▷ 15

Key ▶ **D**

Q3) Which of the following are indications for short-burst oxygen therapy?

  A ▷ Infective exacerbations of COPD

  B ▷ Palliative care

  C ▷ Pre-oxygenation prior to exercise

  D ▷ Breathlessness following exercise

Key ▶ **B**

The role of oxygen therapy

Oxygen is widely available and commonly prescribed in all medical settings. When appropriately administered it reduces both mortality and morbidity in both acute and chronic clinical scenarios. Inappropriate dosing and failure to monitor and adjust treatment can have serious consequences.

Recognising inadequate tissue oxygenation

All human tissue requires oxygen in order to survive. Maintaining an adequate oxygen supply depends upon:

▷ adequate ventilation

▷ appropriate gas exchange

▷ adequate circulatory system to distribute oxygen.

Tissue hypoxia (a lack of oxygen to the tissues) has two patho-physiological mechanisms:

▷ those causing *arterial hypoxaemia* (a lack of oxygen entering the circulatory system). Examples of this include high altitude (a low inspired oxygen partial pressure), alveolar hypoventilation (as seen in sleep apnoea or in opiate overdose), ventilation-perfusion mismatch (acute asthma) or right to left shunts

▷ those causing *failure of the oxygen-haemoglobin transport system*. Examples
of this include inadequate tissue perfusion or low haemoglobin
concentration (as seen in anaemia).

Early recognition of tissue hypoxia is essential to the success of treatment.
Clinical signs can often be non-specific, but include:

▷ dyspnoea
▷ peripheral cyanosis
▷ tachypnoea
▷ altered mental states
▷ arrhythmia.

Clinical measures include assessment of the partial pressure of oxygen in
arterial blood (PaO_2) measured using arterial blood gas (ABG) analysis or the
arterial blood oxygen saturation (SpO_2) measured using pulse oximetry.

Key points

▶ Appropriately prescribed oxygen is helpful in reducing morbidity and
mortality in chronic respiratory disease.
▶ Early recognition of hypoxia is essential in improving the success of
treatment.

Assessment for oxygen therapy

Arterial blood gas analysis

ABG analysis has traditionally been available only in hospital settings, but
with advances in technology it is becoming more widespread in primary
care and community settings, such as community hospitals. Primary care
practitioners without direct access to the test will still need to have an understanding of the interpretation of the results to ensure that appropriate care
is being offered to their patients.

The test procedure is outlined below, followed by more in-depth discussion focusing on the analysis and application to clinical practice.

ABG analysis requires the practitioner to obtain a sample of arterial blood.
This is usually obtained from the radial artery in the wrist as it is close to
the surface and usually has a good collateral circulation, which ensures an
adequate blood supply to the distal tissues during and following the procedure. The sample needs to be analysed immediately (part of the reason that
this test has been predominantly used in secondary care) as the cellular

constituents of the blood remain metabolically active within the sample, which can lead to inaccurate results.

In recent years the test has been developed to enable capillary blood to be obtained from the earlobe, which has fewer risks as it is less invasive than arterial blood sampling.[1] The results obtained between capillary and arterial samples are equitablc.[2]

INTERPRETATION OF ARTERIAL BLOOD GAS ANALYSIS

Analysis of the ABGs is used to determine the patient's ability to maintain normal cell function. Analysis does not routinely measure all gases present in the blood, but usually measures:

▷ pH
▷ $PaCO_2$
▷ SpO_2
▷ PaO_2
▷ HCO_3–
▷ acid/base excess or deficit.

In the UK, the standard unit of measurement is the kilopascal (kPa) with electrolytes being measured in millimoles per litre (mmol/l).

The normal values for each of the parameters are shown in Table 12.1, along with a description of the significance of an abnormal result.

Pulse oximetry

The measurement of the saturation of arterial blood (SpO_2) is a simple, non-invasive measurc that involves placing a small probe onto the patient's finger or carlobe. The probe measures the percentage of haemoglobin (Hb) that is saturated with oxygen.

Oximeters work by sending a source of light from the probe. This light is absorbed by the haemoglobin in differing amounts depending on whether the haemoglobin is saturated with oxygen or not. By calculating the absorption the oximeter can determine the proportion (per cent) of haemoglobin that is oxygenated. The computer within the oximeter is capable of distinguishing pulsatile flow from other more static signals (such as tissue or venous signals) to display only the arterial flow.

Pulse oximeter readings might not be accurate in certain situations:

1 ▷ a reduction in peripheral pulsatile blood flow produced by peripheral vasoconstriction (hypovolaemia, severe hypotension, cold,

230

Table 12.1 ○ *Normal values, parameters and abnormal results*

Parameter	Normal value	Interpretation
PaO_2	11.5–13 kPa	Measurement of partial pressure of oxygen in the blood < 11.5 kPa indicates insufficient oxygen in the blood > 13 kPa indicates excessive oxygen in the blood
pH	7.35–7.45	Measurement of the hydrogen ion concentration in the blood <7.35 indicates acidosis >7.45 indicates alkalosis
$PaCO_2$	4.5–6.0 kPa	Measurement of the partial pressure of carbon dioxide in the blood <6 kPa indicates acidosis >4.5 kPa indicates alkalosis
HCO_3-	22–6 mmol/l	The amount of HCO_3- in the blood <22 mmol/l indicates acidosis >26 mmol/l indicates acidosis
Base excess/ base deficit	-2 ± 2 mmol/l	Base excess is the amount of acid (in mmol/l) required to restore 1 litre of blood to a normal pH of 7.4 Base deficit is the amount of alkali (in mmol/l) required to restore 1 litre of blood to a normal pH of 7.4
SpO_2	93–8%	The percentage of oxygen that is bound to haemoglobin <93% indicates that the level of oxygen saturation is insufficient to meet the needs of the body >98% indicates that the level of oxygen saturation is sufficient to meet the needs of the body

Source: adapted from Simpson.[3]

cardiac failure, some cardiac arrhythmias) or peripheral vascular disease. These result in an inadequate signal for analysis

2 ▷ shivering might cause difficulties in picking up an adequate signal

3 ▷ nail varnish might cause falsely low readings. However, the units are not affected by jaundice, dark skin or anaemia.

Pulse oximetry is useful in providing a fast, non-invasive measurement of oxygen saturation. However, it does not provide the same in-depth clinical information obtained from arterial blood gas analysis and can not detect hypercapnia (increased partial pressure of carbon dioxide).

Hypoxic drive

For a small number of patients with chronic disease, respiration is stimulated by falling oxygen levels rather than the usual trigger of increasing levels of carbon dioxide. This is known as hypoxic drive. Hypoxic drive occurs because the CO_2 levels become permanently elevated and the CO_2 receptors cease responding. For these patients, administering oxygen can actually suppress respiration, increasing hypercapnia. If oxygen therapy is necessary it should be given in a controlled manner.

Symptoms of early hypercapnia, where arterial carbon dioxide pressure, $PaCO_2$, is elevated but not extremely so, include flushed skin, fast pulse, extrasystoles, muscle twitches, hand flaps and possibly a raised blood pressure. In severe hypercapnia (generally $PaCO_2$ greater than $10\,kPa$) symptomatology progresses to disorientation, panic, hyperventilation, convulsions, unconsciousness, and eventually death.

In the short term patients are more at risk from hypoxia than from hypercapnia. The main aim of treatment with oxygen therapy is therefore to correct hypoxia whilst monitoring for signs of hypercapnia.

Key points

▶ Assessment of oxygen level is critical to ensure correct oxygen provision.

▶ Arterial blood gas analysis provides detailed information of the patient's respiratory function.

▶ Pulse oximetry provides a non-invasive method of checking the oxygen saturation of arterial blood. It is readily available and easy to use, but does not give information regarding carbon dioxide levels.

▶ A small number of patients with chronic respiratory disease rely on hypoxia for their respiratory drive. For these patients oxygen therapy may suppress respiration.

▶ In the short term it is more important to correct hypoxia than to restrict oxygen to reduce the risk of hypercapnia.

Oxygen therapy for the acutely breathless patient

Aim of treatment

Oxygen therapy for the acutely breathless patient is aimed at reversing arterial hypoxaemia. The British Thoracic Society's recommendation is that, whenever emergency oxygen is available, there should also be access to pulse oximetry.

Assessment

In some clinical situations ABG analysis might not be immediately available. Pulse oximetry is more readily available and provides a good indication of the degree of hypoxaemia. As with any assessment tool, pulse oximetry or ABG analysis should not be taken in isolation, but should be a component of a complete clinical assessment.

The following have been identified as recommendations for the initiation of oxygen therapy in the acute situation:

▷ cardiac and respiratory arrest
▷ hypoxaemia (PaO_2 < 7.8 kPa, SpO_2 < 90 per cent)
▷ hypotension (systolic blood pressure < 100 mmHg)
▷ low cardiac output and metabolic acidosis (bicarbonate < 18 mmol/l)
▷ respiratory distress (respiratory rate > 24/min).

Initiation of oxygen therapy

It must be remembered that oxygen delivery relies on the patient having and maintaining a patent airway.

In an acute situation the concentration of oxygen delivered might be critical to the success or failure of treatment. The concentration of oxygen given in an acute situation is critical, and inadequate oxygen accounts for more deaths and permanent disability than can be justified considering the relatively low risks of high oxygen concentration prescription.[4]

Selecting a delivery device

A face mask is the preferable method of delivering oxygen to an acutely breathless patient.

A number of different masks are available and should be selected based on the needs of your patient. A cylinder fitted with a high-flow valve will enable the full range to be given.

A *simple oxygen face mask* is a plastic device that fits over a patient's nose and mouth. It delivers oxygen as the patient breathes through either the nose or the mouth. A simple oxygen mask has open side ports that allow room air to enter the mask and dilute the oxygen, as well as allowing exhaled carbon dioxide to leave the containment space.

A simple mask is used to deliver moderate to high concentrations of oxygen. It can deliver from 40 per cent to 60 per cent oxygen at a flow rate of 10–12 l/min.

A *partial rebreather oxygen mask* is similar to a simple face mask; however, the side ports are covered with one-way discs to prevent room air from entering the mask. This mask is called a rebreather because it has a soft plastic reservoir bag connected to the mask that conserves the first third of the patient's exhaled air while the rest escapes through the side ports. This is designed to make use of the carbon dioxide as a respiratory stimulant.

A partial rebreather mask is used to deliver high concentrations of oxygen. It can deliver 70 per cent to 90 per cent oxygen at a flow of 1.58–3.96 gal (6–15 l) per minute.

A *non-rebreather oxygen mask* is similar to a simple face mask but has multiple one-way valves in the side ports. These valves prevent room air from entering the mask but allow exhaled air to leave the mask. It has a reservoir bag like a partial rebreather mask but the reservoir bag has a one-way valve that prevents exhaled air from entering the reservoir. This allows larger concentrations of oxygen to collect in the reservoir bag for the patient to inhale.

A non-rebreather mask is used to deliver high-flow oxygen. It can deliver 90 per cent to 100 per cent oxygen at a flow of 15 l/min.

A *Venturi oxygen mask* is similar to a simple face mask but incorporates an interchangeable Venturi which ensures that specific proportions of oxygen and room air are mixed to deliver a fixed concentration of oxygen (the fraction of inspired oxygen – FiO_2). Table 12.2 below shows the number of litres of oxygen and the corresponding oxygen concentration delivered to the patient. However, it is always advisable to check this with any mask and equipment you use.

Table 12.2 ○ *Oxygen concentration*

l/min	FiO_2 (%)
2	24
4	28
6	31
8	35
15	50

The following flow charts provide guidelines for oxygen prescription in acute scenarios.

Figure 12.1 ○ *Oxygen prescription guidance*[1]

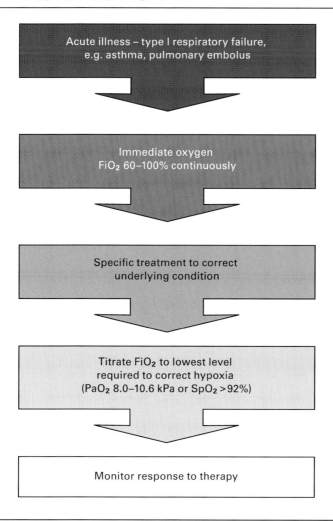

Acute illness – type I respiratory failure,
e.g. asthma, pulmonary embolus

Immediate oxygen
FiO_2 60–100% continuously

Specific treatment to correct
underlying condition

Titrate FiO_2 to lowest level
required to correct hypoxia
(PaO_2 8.0–10.6 kPa or SpO_2 >92%)

Monitor response to therapy

Source: reproduced by kind permission of Education for Health.

Monitoring response to treatment

▷ If possible ABG analysis or pulse oximetry should be carried out before oxygen therapy is commenced.

▷ ABG analysis or pulse oximetry should be measured within 2 hours of starting oxygen therapy and alterations made to treatment to ensure an adequate response (defined as PaO_2 >7.8 kPa or SpO_2 >90 per cent).

▷ Patients at risk of arrhythmia or respiratory failure should be monitored continuously.

Figure 12.2 ○ *Oxygen prescription guidance*[2]

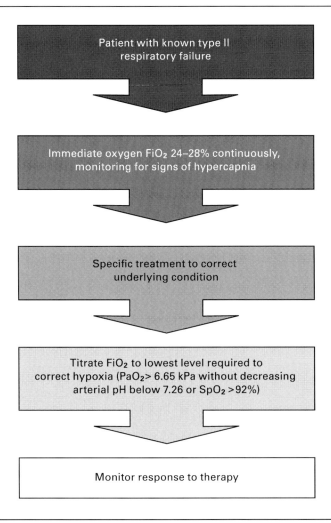

Patient with known type II respiratory failure

Immediate oxygen FiO_2 24–28% continuously, monitoring for signs of hypercapnia

Specific treatment to correct underlying condition

Titrate FiO_2 to lowest level required to correct hypoxia ($PaO_2 >$ 6.65 kPa without decreasing arterial pH below 7.26 or $SpO_2 >$92%)

Monitor response to therapy

Source: reproduced by kind permission of Education for Health.

Stopping treatment

Oxygen therapy should be stopped when the patient is able to maintain adequate oxygenation whilst breathing room air.

Key points

▶ In the acutely breathless patient oxygen therapy is aimed at reversing arterial hypoxaemia. The following are recommendations for the initiation of oxygen therapy:

▷ cardiac and respiratory arrest

▷ hypoxaemia (PaO_2 <7.8 kPa, SpO_2 <90 per cent)

▷ hypotension (systolic blood pressure <100 mmHg)

▷ low cardiac output and metabolic acidosis (bicarbonate <18 mmol/l)

▷ respiratory distress (respiratory rate >24/min).

▶ The appropriate delivery device should be selected to deliver the appropriate percentage of oxygen. A summary of the available devices is shown on Table 12.3.

▶ For patients with type I respiratory failure oxygen should be started at 60–100% and titrated downwards to the lowest level required to correct hypoxia.

▶ For patients with type II respiratory failure oxygen should be started at 24–28% and titrated upwards to the lowest level required to correct hypoxia.

▶ Monitoring of patients receiving oxygen should take place at regular intervals and for those at risk of arrhythmia or respiratory failure it should be constant.

▶ Treatment should be stopped when a patient is able to maintain oxygenation whilst breathing room air.

Table 12.3 ○ *Available delivery devices*

Device	Flow rate (l/min)	% FiO_2
Simple face mask	10–12	40–60
Partial rebreather mask	6–15	70–90
Non-rebreather mask	15 l	90–100
Venturi mask	2–15	24–50

Oxygen therapy in chronic breathlessness

Aim of treatment

Oxygen therapy for people with chronic breathlessness is aimed at reducing symptoms and improving quality of life. Oxygen for chronic hypoxic COPD improves life expectancy. The first trial conducted by the Medical Research Council (MRC)[5] showed that 15 hours of oxygen per day increased 5-year survival from 25 per cent to 41 per cent. The NOTT trial (Nocturnal Oxygen

Therapy Trial)[6] showed that the use of oxygen continuously was beneficial (mean time of use 17.7 hours) but use for less than 12 hours a day was of no benefit.

Oxygen delivered for this group of patients is known as home oxygen therapy. There are different methods by which home oxygen can be delivered, depending on the needs of the individual patient. All patients should be assessed on an individual basis to ensure that they receive the most appropriate dose and delivery method to meet their needs.

Short-burst and ambulatory oxygen therapy (oxygen cylinders)

Oxygen cylinders provide *short-burst oxygen therapy*, usually for periods of 10–20 minutes to relieve dyspnoea.

Cylinders are also used in the provision of *ambulatory oxygen therapy*, which is the continuous supply of supplemental oxygen during exercise or activity.

Short-burst oxygen therapy is provided by cylinders for home use. In the UK these cylinders contain 1360 litres of oxygen, which at a flow rate of 2 l/min provides approximately 11 hours of oxygen.[7] The cylinder valve allows the oxygen flow rate to be regulated at either a medium flow rate (2 l/min) or a high flow rate (4 l/min).

Ambulatory oxygen can be delivered using smaller, portable oxygen cylinders. These cylinders typically contain 300 litres and at a flow rate of 2 l/min will provide approximately two hours of oxygen. Unfortunately many patients find these cylinders cumbersome and carrying the additional weight can cancel out the benefits obtained from using oxygen whilst active. Newer, lightweight cylinders are available. Portable liquid oxygen cylinders containing a litre of liquid oxygen provide oxygen for 8–10 days (at a flow rate of 2 l/min) and are filled from a reservoir in the patient's home. Oxygen-conserving devices, which extend the life of portable cylinders, are more widely available since the changes to the prescribing arrangements.

The oxygen system most suitable for the individual patient should now be available, with device selection based on assessment of individual needs.

Indications for prescribing oxygen therapy via cylinders

Short-burst oxygen therapy has traditionally been used for:

▷ pre-oxygenation prior to exercise
▷ breathlessness during recovery following exercise
▷ control of breathlessness during rest
▷ palliative care

▷ after an exacerbation of COPD to bridge the time to full oxygen assessment.

Despite the widespread prescription of short-burst oxygen therapy there is no adequate evidence available to support its use pre- or post-exercise or in the control of breathlessness at rest.[8,9]

Short-burst oxygen therapy should however be considered for intermittent, episodic breathlessness that does not respond to other treatments in the following circumstances:

▷ patients with severe chronic obstructive pulmonary disease
▷ patients with interstitial lung disease
▷ patients with heart failure
▷ palliative care.

Short-burst oxygen therapy should only be prescribed where there is documented evidence of an improvement in breathlessness and/or exercise tolerance.[10]

Ambulatory oxygen therapy should be considered for patients receiving long-term oxygen therapy who have remained mobile and leave the home on a regular basis. Patients not receiving long-term oxygen therapy but with evidence of exercise desaturation should also be considered for ambulatory oxygen. Ambulatory oxygen is not recommended for patients with chronic heart failure.[10]

Long-term oxygen therapy (oxygen concentrators)

Long-term oxygen therapy is prescribed for people requiring continuous oxygen therapy at home to correct chronic hypoxaemia. Long-term oxygen therapy is provided via an oxygen concentrator. Oxygen concentrators 'sieve' room air, removing nitrogen, to provide 95 per cent oxygen. At higher flow rates the oxygen concentration drops to between 85–90 per cent.[7]

The oxygen flow rate must be sufficient to correct the hypoxaemia. Long-term oxygen therapy is usually given for 15 hours per day including night-time in recognition of the presence of worsening hypoxaemia during sleep.

Assessment for long-term oxygen therapy

Long-term oxygen therapy should only be prescribed to patients who meet the following criteria when clinically stable (defined as the absence of an exacerbation of the underlying lung disease for a minimum of 5 weeks):

▷ PaO$_2$ of 7.3 kPa when breathing room air, measured by ABG analysis on at least two occasions not less than 3 weeks apart

or

▷ PaO$_2$ of 7.3–8.0 kPa when breathing room air, measured by ABG analysis on at least two occasions not less than 3 weeks apart together with the presence of one of the following:

- secondary polycythaemia
- clinical or echocardiography evidence of pulmonary hypertension.

Selecting a delivery device

For many patients receiving oxygen therapy for chronic breathlessness, selection of a delivery device is guided by patient preference. Most patients receiving long-term oxygen therapy use nasal cannulae.

A nasal cannula is a narrow, flexible plastic tube that delivers oxygen through the nostrils of patients using nose breathing. It fits over the patient's ears and is brought together under the chin by a sliding connector that holds the device in place. Two slightly curved prongs fit into the front portion of a patient's nostrils.

A nasal cannula is used to deliver low concentrations of oxygen. It can deliver from 24 per cent to 40 per cent oxygen at a flow rate of 1–6 l/min; however, the concentration varies depending on whether the patient is nose or mouth breathing.

The advantages of using nasal cannulae, particularly in the delivery of long-term oxygen therapy, lie in their comfort for patients. They are simple, unobtrusive and do not restrict day-to-day activities such as eating, drinking or talking. However, they can cause drying and soreness inside the nose. This can be a big problem for patients and, while soreness around the ears and cheeks can be alleviated, this is sometimes a cause of non-adherence. There is a risk of pressure sores developing, particularly behind the ears and around the nose. These can be avoided by the use of pads or non-petroleum-based moisturising cream.

Monitoring response to treatment

All patients receiving home oxygen therapy should be under the care of a specialist team who manage the home oxygen service for each Primary Care Team. This team is responsible for reviewing the efficacy and appropriateness of the treatment.

Key points

▶ Patients requiring oxygen therapy for chronic disease should be assessed by a specialist team.

▶ Oxygen can be prescribed for use as either short burst, ambulatory or long-term oxygen therapy.

▶ Short-burst and ambulatory oxygen is delivered by oxygen cylinder.

▶ Long-term oxygen therapy is delivered via an oxygen concentrator.

▶ If used appropriately long-term oxygen therapy is known to increase life expectancy.

The home oxygen therapy service

In 2006 a radical overhaul of the home oxygen therapy service was rolled out across the UK. The service was designed to standardise the provision of home oxygen and to ensure that all patients have equal access to the full range of oxygen delivery technologies.

The new service has seen the UK divided into ten oxygen regions. Each region has a single oxygen supplier, who provides the oxygen service for all patients in that area.

Patients are assessed by a specialist team who determine the individual needs of the patient. The team is responsible for follow-up and monitoring of each patient.

In general practice, a GP can still prescribe short-burst oxygen for use in palliative care or emergency oxygen for short-term use prior to full oxygen assessment. For patients requiring other forms of oxygen therapy, referral to the specialist team is necessary.

Further self-assessment

1) Consider the following scenarios:

A ▷ An 87-year-old smoker with severe COPD requiring long-term oxygen therapy

B ▷ A 57-year-old retired surgeon who suffers from cluster headaches and believes that short-burst oxygen helps these

C ▷ A patient who is terminally ill with mesothelioma
  For each scenario consider:
  ■ Is oxygen indicated?
  ■ Who can or should make this decision?

Figure 12.3 ○ *Home Oxygen Order Form (HOOF)*

Home Oxygen Order Form (HOOF)
Please read the accompanying guidance notes before completing this order form

NHS

1

Title:	Gender: M / F
Surname:	
First name:	
Date of Birth:	
Patient Tel. Number:	
Mobile Tel. No:	
Patient NHS No:	
Patient Hospital No:	

Is this a Paediatric order?   Yes ☐   No ☐

Has Patient consent been obtained   Yes ☐   No ☐

2

Patient's address (use label where available)

Post Code:

Is this the permanent home address?   Yes ☐   No ☐
(if no please give more details in 6 to assist the oxygen supplier)
or   **School / Work address give additional information in 13**

Carer's Name:

Carer Tel. Number:

3

Clinical contact for enquiries (GP practice or assessment team):

Name:

Tel. No: Fax:

E-mail:

4

Hospital address and Code:

Post Code:

5   Patient's GPs practice (main branch) address:

Tel. No: Fax:

E-Mail:

PCT / LHB Name:

6   If this is a **Holiday Order** give additional information in 13 below

7 LONG TERM OXYGEN THERAPY

Litres / minute:

Hours / day:

Nasal cannulae   Yes ☐   No ☐

Mask   (__ __ %)

Humidification   Yes ☐   No ☐

8 AMBULATORY

Litres / minute:

Hours / day:

Initial two month's supply Yes ☐   No ☐

Light weight option   Yes ☐   No ☐

9 SHORT BURST OXYGEN

Litres / minute:

Hours / day:

Nasal cannulae   Yes ☐   No ☐

Mask   (__ __ %)

10 EMERGENCY ORDER

Duration of emergency order ___ days (max 3 days)

11 HOSPITAL DISCHARGE ORDER

Is next day response required   Yes ☐   No ☐

Is this temporary prior to stable assessment for LTOT   Yes ☐   No ☐

Ward tel. no.

Please complete boxes 7 or 9 for service required.

12 Date of planned assessment / order review date

13 Additional information for the home oxygen service supplier

14 Clinical information
Clinical code: __ __

On NIV   Yes ☐   No ☐

On CPAP   Yes ☐   No ☐

Conserving device contra indicated   ☐

15 I confirm that I am a registered healthcare professional

Signature:	Date:	Pin:
Name (Print):	Position:	
E-mail:	Tel. No:	Fax No:

Original to oxygen supplier FAX Number.. Copies to: PCT / LHB, GP, Trust Clinical Lead for home oxygen, Patient's record. It is an offence to falsify the details on this form. The NHS Counter Fraud Service will pursue all sanctions, including appropriate legal action, against any persons committing fraud.

ADVISORY NOTES: Please give full contact details so that the oxygen supplier can contact you to resolve queries.
This form should NOT be used where patients are experiencing problems with a current supply.
Please use supplier 24/7 helpline to report these.

Box 3: Please indicate name of Consultant (if applicable) and details of clinical contact.

Box 5: You **must** complete Primary Care Trust (PCT) / or Local Health Board (LHB) Wales. The oxygen supplier will be invoicing the PCT/ LHB; therefore you should take care to enter the correct details so that payment can be made by the correct PCT / LHB (payment is based on the location of the patient's GP's main surgery, not the patient's address). **You must** also send a copy order to the PCT / LHB for audit purposes.

Box 6: Holiday order: If a patient requires oxygen at a UK holiday destination, at school or work, a secondary order form is required to provide oxygen in a location other than the patient's home. Please ensure this order provides the correct delivery address, information about access / named person receiving equipment and, where appropriate, start and completion date of holiday. Note that a patient on holiday may require a different service.

Consent: Patient consent is needed to provide personal information to the supplier to enable delivery of the service to be made - that is for the supplier to hold certain personal information about the patient. If consent has not been obtained, the supplier will be in breach of the Data Protection Act 1998.

Box 7: An **LTOT** request will **not** automatically include provision of oxygen for use outside the home. If this is needed please also complete box 8.

Box 8: Ambulatory oxygen: **Adults and older children:** Initial assessment must be performed in accordance with the clinical component of the home oxygen service. A 2 month assessment period is required so that hours of usage can be determined. Therefore it is suggested that initially 1-2 hours per day is ordered, allowing 7-14 hours of oxygen per week. If the usage changes then the hours per day can be increased or decreased by completing a new order.

Infants: Children on LTOT will usually need ambulatory oxygen. An initial order of 3-4 hours per day is suggested, with review after 2 months.

Box 9: Short burst oxygen: This will normally be ordered for symptomatic relief or breathlessness, in patients using oxygen for less than 2 hours per day. A static source of oxygen will be provided. Nasal cannulae will be appropriate for short burst oxygen. The usual flow rate is 2-4 litres per minute using a 24-28% mask.

Box 10: Emergency supply: Clinicians should order this service only where a patient requires an urgent supply of oxygen and has no oxygen supply at home. The supplier is required to deliver this service within 4 hours of receipt of the order. It should not be ordered for more than three days. To avoid the emergency tariff being charged longer than necessary, clinical staff will need to ensure that a second HOOF is completed for non-emergency supply at the same time, or as soon as possible after the emergency order is made. The emergency service should not be ordered where a patient has problems with an existing supply or has a back-up cylinder. **The patient or carer should be advised to contact the supplier 24/7 helpline.**

Box 11: Hospital discharge: When arranging a supply of oxygen to support discharge, please give a contact name and ward telephone number and carer's telephone number in boxes 2 & 3 so that the oxygen supplier can gain access to the patient's home. If discharge planning has not allowed sufficient time for a viable 3 day response, a next day supply of oxygen can be provided (tick yes in Box 11) to prevent delayed discharge. If a 6 week temporary supply of oxygen is required prior to the stable LTOT assessment, this should be indicated in box 12.

Box 12: Order review date: must be stated if patient is awaiting second assessment for LTOT or when ambulatory oxygen 2 month assessment period ends or if emergency oxygen has been ordered.

Box 13: Please note any special needs e.g. language or disabilities.

Box 14: Clinical codes: (As suggested by BTS)

01	Chronic obstructive pulmonary disease (COPD)	02	Pulmonary vascular disease
03	Severe chronic asthma	04	Primary pulmonary hypertension
05	Interstitial lung disease	06	Pulmonary malignancy
07	Cystic fibrosis	08	Palliative care
09	Bronchiectasis (Not cystic fibrosis)	10	Non-pulmonary palliative care
11	Chronic heart failure	12	Paediatric interstitial lung disease
13	Chronic neonatal lung disease	14	Neuromuscular disease
15	Paediatric cardiac disease	16	Neurodisability
17	Chest wall disease	18	Other primary respiratory disorder
19	Obstructive sleep apnoea syndrome	20	Other conditions

Service categories:

	SERVICE CATEGORIES	RESPONSE TIME	DURATION OF PRESCRIPTION	AMBULATORY
CC1	Emergency	4 Hours	Up to 3 days	Not applicable
CC2	i) On discharge pending formal assessment	Next day between 8.00am and 05.00pm	Up to 4/5 weeks until the patient is able to be formally assessed	Not applicable
	ii) Short burst	3 Days	Long term	Not applicable
CC3	Long term oxygen therapy	3 Days	Long term	Not applicable
CC4	Long term oxygen therapy and standard ambulatory supply	3 Days	Long term	Yes
CC5	Standard ambulatory supply only	3 Days	Long term	Yes
CC6	Long term oxygen therapy and lightweight ambulatory supply	3 Days	Long term	Yes
CC7	Lightweight ambulatory supply only	3 Days	Long term	Yes

Supplier 24/7 helplines, fax numbers and areas:

	Tel:	Fax:	
Air Products	0800 373580	0800 214709	North West, Yorks and Humberside, Leics, Northants & Rutland,Trent, Birmingham and Black Country, Shrops & Staffs, West Midlands, Wales, North East London , North West & Central London, South West Peninsula, Dorset & Somerset, Avon, Glos & Wilts.
Allied Respiratory	0500 823773	0800 781 4610	SW & SE London, Thames Valley, Hants & IOW, Kent & Medway, Surrey & Sussex
BOC Vitalair	0800 136603	0800 169 9989	Beds & Herts, Essex, Norfolk, Suffolk & Cambs.
Linde	0808 2020999	0191 497 4340	Co. Durham, Northumberland, Tyne and Wear, and Tees Valley.

- What investigations are necessary prior to prescribing oxygen?
- If oxygen is indicated what steps would you take to ensure that your patient is supplied appropriately.

2) For those patients in Q1 that you would prescribe oxygen for, complete a Home Oxygen Order Form (HOOF).

Further resources

NHS Home Oxygen Service information • **www.homeoxygen.nhs.uk**.

Further reading

Bateman N T, Leach R M. ABC of oxygen: acute oxygen therapy *British Medical Journal* 1998; **317**: 798–801.

British Thoracic Society Emergency Oxygen Guideline Group. Guideline for emergency oxygen use in adult patients *Thorax* 2008; **63(6)**.

British Thoracic Society Standards of Care Committee. Managing passengers with respiratory disease planning air travel *Thorax* 2002; **57**: 289–304.

References

1 • Dunn L, Connolly C. Diagnostic investigations. In: G Cox (ed.). *Respiratory Nursing* London: Baillière Tindall, 2001, pp. 59–79.

2 • Woodrow P. Arterial blood gas analysis *Nursing Standard* 2004; **18(21)**: 45–52.

3 • Simpson H. Interpretation of arterial blood gases: a clinical guide for nurses *British Journal of Nursing* 2004; **13(9)**: 522–8.

4 • Bateman N T, Leach R M. ABC of Oxygen: Acute oxygen therapy *British Medical Journal* 1998; **317**: 798–801.

5 • Medical Research Council, Working Party. Long term domiciliary oxygen therapy in chronic hypoxic cor pulmonale complicating chronic bronchitis and emphysema *Lancet* 1981; **1**: 681–6.

6 • Nocturnal Oxygen Therapy Trial (NOTT) Group. Continuous or nocturnal oxygen therapy in hypoxaemic COPD. A clinical trial *Annals of Internal Medicine* 1980; **93**: 391–8.

7 • Rees P J, Dudley F. ABC of Oxygen: provision of oxygen at home *British Medical Journal* 1998; **317**: 935–8.

8 • Stevenson N J, Calverley P M A. Effect of oxygen on recovery from maximal exercise in patients with chronic obstructive pulmonary disease *Thorax* 2004; **59**: 668–72.

9 • Smith A A, Crawford A, MacRae K D, *et al.* Oxygen supplementation before or after submaximal exercise in patients with chronic obstructive pulmonary disease *Thorax* 2003; **58**: 670–3.

10 • BTS Working Group on Home Oxygen Therapy Services. *Clinical Component for the Home Oxygen Therapy Service in England and Wales* London: BTS, 2006, www.brit-thoracic. org.uk/Portals/0/Clinical%20Information/Home%20Oxygen%20Service/clinical%20 adultoxygenjan06.pdf [accessed January 2009].

Evaluating quality of care

13

Simon Gregory

Introduction

It is every practitioner's personal and professional responsibility to ensure that he or she provides an appropriate standard of care. But what is an appropriate standard of care and how do we know that we are providing it? For some it is the standard of care you would want provided for a relative or close friend. For others it is care above the legal cut-off according to the Bolam principle. The Bolam principle states that the doctor is not liable for his or her diagnosis or treatment, or refusal to give information to the patient, if he or she follows a responsible body of medical opinion.[1] Yet neither of these truly indicates what 'quality of care' is or for that matter what high-quality care is.

Chapter aims and learning outcomes

In this curriculum guide we have sought to support your understanding of respiratory medicine in primary care. As a general practitioner (GP) you will be expected to lead a team and to ensure that you and that team provide a satisfactory standard of care. In this chapter we consider how you might gather information to direct, evaluate and benchmark the care you provide. We will consider:

▶ clinical governance
▶ Evidence-Based Practice
   ▷ guidelines
   ▷ protocols
   ▷ audit
▶ contracts and regulation
▶ continuing professional development.

You should use this chapter to reflect on how you will apply that which you have learned from this curriculum guide and how you will continually review and update your learning throughout your professional life. The RCGP curriculum on which GP specialty training is founded is itself based on six core competences. These six are variously expressed when considering each general practice situation. In particular in evaluating the quality of care you provide to patients or practices with respiratory disorders you might want to consider these competences. For example, how does your practice balance person-centred care (individual care) with community orientation?

Initial self-assessment

You are newly appointed as a GP in a salaried role in an inner-city practice. Your next patient is a 47-year-old ex-smoker with a chronic cough; he attends with his lung function test print-out (spirometry including reversibility) that has been performed by a healthcare assistant in the practice earlier in the day. The patient is concerned about his cough and the effect on his work and home life. Consider the antecedents to this consultation and how you will interpret this print-out in the light of his concerns. Use the following questions to assist your consideration. It is suggested that you make notes of your answers in order to compare them with your learning after reading this chapter. You might wish to refer to Chapters 4 and 8 (on asthma and chronic obstructive pulmonary disease [COPD]) to inform your thinking.

▷ Why was the spirometry performed?
▷ How was the person performing it trained and assessed?
▷ Is the equipment fully functioning and calibrated according to the manufacturer's instructions?
▷ How was reversibility assessed?
▷ Can you trust the result?
▷ How would you interpret it?
▷ How will it inform your conclusions about a diagnosis?
▷ What will you tell your patient?
▷ What will guide your treatment choices and decisions?
▷ Having looked at the print-out do you identify any personal learning needs?
▷ If so how will you address them?

Clinical governance

The concept of clinical governance arose from the NHS Plan.[2] This placed a 'duty of quality' on all NHS organisations: a duty it could be said that already existed for professionals through medical ethics or even the Hippocratic

Oath but that now has to be demonstrated. It has been described as 'trying to ensure that … patients get the best possible, and affordable, care … a philosophy … that demands personal responsibility for the totality of the experience that patients receive'.[3] It is important that this is a philosophy and not a checklist. It includes many elements (Box 13.1).

Box 13.1 ○ *'The ten commandments of clinical governance'*[4]

1 Evidence-Based Practice with the infrastructure to support it.
2 Good practice, ideas and innovations systematically disseminated.
3 Quality improvement programmes, for example clinical audit.
4 High-quality data to monitor clinical care.
5 Clinical risk reduction programmes.
6 Adverse events detected and openly investigated; the lessons learnt promptly applied.
7 Lessons for clinical practice systematically learnt from complaints made by patients.
8 Problems of poor clinical performance recognised at an early stage and dealt with.
9 All professional development programmes reflect principles of clinical governance.
10 Leadership skill development at clinical team level.

Source: van Zwanenberg and Edwards.[4]

For these elements to be truly present requires a positive culture that encourages reflection, constructive criticism and development, and requires each individual to seek to achieve the best. This does not mean that we will all always deliver the best; it is likely that for both individuals and for organisations there will be a normal distribution of the quality of care we provide. Good clinical governance systems should shift this distribution to the right. As a clinical leader in your practice you will need to ensure sound clinical governance of the practice is in place. This might include ensuring appropriate, sound systems, suitable employment practices, training and appraisal of staff, organisational systems that include clinical and managerial input, and the practice's quality assurance systems.

To ensure that the organisation in which doctors work meets the necessary standards it is essential to assess their own clinical practice and for the organisation to assess itself. This might involve a baseline assessment (such as against *Standards for Better Health*)[5] or a cycle of quality assessment and improvement (such as the RCGP's former accreditation system, Quality Team Development, or its proposed replacement, Practice Accreditation, which is currently being piloted).

Whatever approach is used it is worthwhile grounding any assessment in the domains of *Standards for Better Health* since these are an NHS requirement. These are: safety, clinical and cost-effectiveness, governance (including corporate and clinical), patient focus, accessible and responsive care, care environment and amenities, and public health.

Evidence-Based Practice

Evidence-Based Practice is talked of as if it is something new. It is not: some attribute its philosophy to mid-nineteenth-century Paris. In reality doctors have been seeking to practise according to the available evidence for centuries. However, the use of the phrase 'best-evidence practice' has been in common parlance since the 1990s. Evidence-Based Practice can be defined as 'the conscientious, explicit and judicious use of current best evidence in making decisions about the care of individual patients'.[6] Indeed the same authors suggest that 'it's about integrating individual clinical expertise and the best external evidence'. Approaches to Evidence-Based Practice are now taught at medical school and in postgraduate training. As GPs we practise holistic medicine and do so with the individual patient as our primary focus at the time of the consultation. To do so is about more than simply finding and evaluating the available evidence. It is about the synthesis of factors using our clinical expertise, combining the clinical state and circumstances and the patient's preferences and actions with the best available, evaluated research evidence (Figure 13.1). As GPs we should combine these factors and present the information to our patients in a form that enables the patient to make an informed treatment choice and where necessary to give informed consent.

It is questionable how much we truly encourage informed participation of our patients. Many patients do not dare seek an active part in decision making, true; however, do we truly encourage this participation? Perhaps our own innumeracy regarding risk and its explanation makes accessing and sharing this information daunting. Perhaps we sometimes therefore project the 'illusion of certainty'.[7] Once we have evaluated evidence we should recognise where doubt still exists, and also that the evidence might be later disproved. But this should not decry the value of the evidence or act as justification for poor practice.

Patients are becoming ever more informed. Many now glean information from websites of varying accuracy and quality before they consult healthcare professionals. Whilst healthcare systems need to ensure that patients can access clean, clear information, professionals need to adapt to this new breed of informed patient. It might be that we reflect and interpret the infor-

Figure 13.1 ○ *A holistic approach to Evidence-Based Practice*

Clinical state and
circumstances

Patients' preferences
and actions

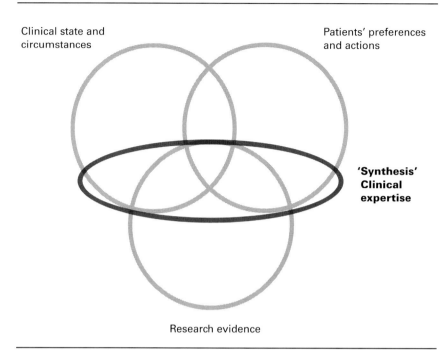

**'Synthesis'
Clinical
expertise**

Research evidence

mation or that we need to sensitively contradict it, or on occasions that the patient is better informed than we are.

A detailed analysis of how to evaluate and apply evidence is beyond the scope of this chapter. In simple terms this is about finding and appraising evidence, ensuring that you and your organisation have the capacity to apply the evidence and ensuring that research is appropriately transformed into practice. Typically such appraisal would include considering the research methods, the outcomes and the application (or resulting health-related decisions).

It is a sad reality that only a small proportion of the published literature is of high quality and there is a paucity of good-quality research. Recommended strategies by which to address this are to employ robust search strategies and to use specialised databases, perhaps with the help of a good librarian. Sometimes you may wish to make reference to original literature but commonly we will use reviews (especially systematic reviews) and guidelines. Even these we should evaluate and consider their provenance, accuracy and pertinence. The first guidelines to make a truly effective national impact were the original British Thoracic Society Asthma Guidelines (1990). These guidelines dramatically altered clinical practice in the UK and further afield. Yet these were largely based on consensus rather than robust evidence. They have since been replaced with newer and more robust guidelines. The BTS/

Figure 13.2 ○ **Levels of evidence**

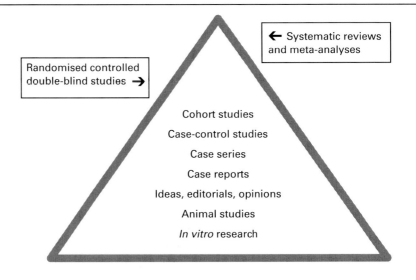

SIGN guidelines are based on a hierarchy of evidence. However, the pro-liferation of guidelines has perhaps lessened their impact as we now suffer from guideline overload. Perhaps the most useful sources are systematic reviews and national guidelines such as produced by Cochrane, Clinical Evidence, the Scottish Intercollegiate Guidelines Network (SIGN) and the National Institute for Health and Clinical Excellence (NICE). In considering these reviews it is worthwhile considering the grades of evidence used for their recommendations (Table 13.1 and Figure 13.2) and the independence and composition of the group. Are they relevant to primary care? Have they been influenced by sponsorship such as from pharmaceutical companies or by pressure groups? Do they actually make clinical sense or is there an immediate incongruity for you?

There is then a difficulty considering the legal implications of guidelines and of following them or not. However good a guideline (even from NICE) it does not have automatic legal effect. Here again we fall back upon the Bolam principle,[1] but a widely accepted authoritative guideline can provide a good defence in the hands of a good barrister. And if you chose not to use a guideline you might need to justify why not.

The application of guidelines is difficult. Even once you decide which ones to use there will be more than it is humanly possible to remember, and as doctors we typically apply fuzzy logic and leap to an appropriate action

Table 13.1 ○ **Grading system for recommendations in evidence-based guidelines**

Levels of evidence	
1++	High-quality meta-analyses, systematic reviews of RCTs (randomised controlled trials), or RCTs with a very low risk of bias
1+	Well-conducted meta-analyses, systematic reviews of RCTs, or RCTs with a low risk of bias
1−	Meta-analyses, systematic reviews or RCTs, or RCTs with a high risk of bias
2++	High-quality systematic reviews of case-control or cohort studies or high-quality case-control or cohort studies with a very low risk of confounding, bias or chance and a high probability that the relationship is causal
2+	Well-conducted case-control or cohort studies with a low risk of confounding, bias or chance and a moderate probability that the relationship is causal
2−	Case-control or cohort studies with a high risk of confounding, bias or chance and a significant risk that the relationship is not causal
3	Non-analytic studies, e.g. case reports, case series
4	Expert opinion
Grades of recommendations	
A	At least one meta-analysis, systematic review, or RCT rated as 1++ and directly applicable to the target population or a systematic review of RCTs or a body of evidence consisting principally of studies rated as 1+ directly applicable to the target population and demonstrating overall consistency of results
B	A body of evidence including studies rated as 2++ directly applicable to the target population and demonstrating overall consistency of results or extrapolated evidence from studies rated as 1++ or 1+
C	A body of evidence including studies rated as 2+ directly applicable to the target population and demonstrating overall consistency of results or extrapolated evidence from studies rated as 2++
D	Evidence level 3 or 4 or extrapolated evidence from studies rated as 2+

Source: Harbour R, Miller J. A new system for grading recommendations in evidence based guidelines *British Medical Journal* 2001; **323(7308)**: 334–6. Reproduced with permission from the BMJ Publishing Group.

rather than following algorithms. It is therefore worthwhile to organise your practice in such a way as to encourage application and ready access. This might be by keeping paper copies readily accessible or by linking to them from an intranet, or perhaps even using a good search engine. Another approach is to agree as a primary healthcare team which topics to focus on and to develop local protocols that apply the guidelines to your local circumstances, including which drugs you have in your formulary (e.g. which inhaler devices) and what tests and referral options are available.

The final word on the use of guidelines goes to Lady Thatcher during the Scott Inquiry (the 'Arms to Iraq' affair):[8]

Lady Thatcher: 'They are guidelines. … They are expected to be followed.'

Ms Baxendale QC: 'They are expected to be followed?'

Lady Thatcher: 'That is why we have them, but they are guidelines, they are not a strict interpretation that you would get of a legal system. That is why they are guidelines.'

Ms Baxendale QC: 'I do not think there is any suggestion that they were the law, but I just want to understand whether you thought they needed to be followed.'

Lady Thatcher: 'Of course they need to be followed. They need to be followed for what they are, guidelines.'

We can see that even the Iron Lady sees guidelines as containing some element of ambiguity.

Audit

Audit is the systematic, critical analysis of the quality of medical care. It is a well-established tool used by many practices to improve the quality of their clinical care and practice organisation. Audit can be clinical or non-clinical and is frequently multidisciplinary. Undertaken properly it can be a very effective agent for lasting change. Figures 13.3 and 13.4 show the steps in this process. Figure 13.3 shows a simple approach to audit and Figure 13.4 how NICE has built on this to encourage ongoing development. Audit is often referred to as the audit cycle in order to highlight the need to repeat the process. If audit has successful outcomes of quality improvement then perhaps a helix would be a better geometric description. The new General Medical Services (nGMS) contract[9] brought with it the Quality and Outcomes Framework (QOF) (see below). This has led to considerable activity in the area of data collection but this has not necessarily turned into effective audit. Indeed the QOF covers so vast a range of clinical and non-clinical areas that we could not be reasonably expected to audit all of it. The QOF may highlight areas in which your practice could improve the care it offers but other factors such as new developments, errors and even personal interests may also act as triggers.

Figure 13.3 ○ *Steps in the audit process*

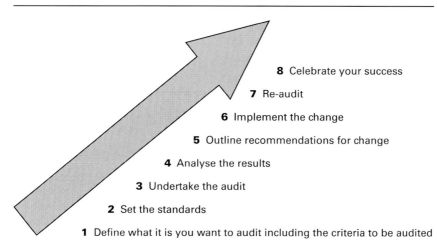

8 Celebrate your success

7 Re-audit

6 Implement the change

5 Outline recommendations for change

4 Analyse the results

3 Undertake the audit

2 Set the standards

1 Define what it is you want to audit including the criteria to be audited

---

Source: copyright Janet Corbett, Chief Pharmacist, Milton Keynes Primary Care Trust.

Figure 13.4 ○ *The stages of clinical audit*

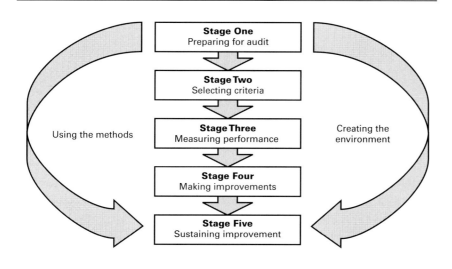

Stage One
Preparing for audit

Stage Two
Selecting criteria

Using the methods

Stage Three
Measuring performance

Creating the environment

Stage Four
Making improvements

Stage Five
Sustaining improvement

Source: © Ashmore S (ed.). *Principles for Best Practice in Clinical Audit* Oxford: Radcliffe Publishing, 2004. Reproduced with the permission of the copyright holder.[10]

Audits take time and energy. It is important that the practice culture is supportive of evaluating the quality of care you deliver and therefore supportive of audit. It takes time to perform audits and it is essential that it is provided. For audits to be performed there needs to be good support, such as help with searches and with implementing changes. Furthermore there needs to be a culture in which openness and creativity are encouraged. There should be a 'no blame' approach, with reporting of errors encouraged without undue fear of blame. If an audit is to have a positive impact as much effort must be devoted to implementing changes as to the data collection, and such change should be welcomed as the antidote to stagnation.

Significant event review

The supporting material for the nGMS[9] refers to significant event review (SER) as an extension of audit activity. It is the discussion of cases and events and learning through reflection and discussion. Like audit it is important to complete the process and where necessary implement changes. Advice on how to implement SER can be found in an RCGP Occasional Paper.[11] The principles are essentially similar to those of audit. Here the significant event is the trigger for the review (audit) and the review process follows the stages of the audit process. Whilst it is encouraging that SER is rewarded within the QOF, the areas that it focuses on are rather limited and the learning points might be similarly limited. Greater benefits can be achieved by broadening the scope of significant events reviewed and ensuring that these are discussed within a supportive, 'no blame' culture. For example, you might wish to consider a patient who has recently been admitted to hospital with severe acute asthma and review his or her pre-admission care to see whether the admission was avoidable.

Quality and Outcomes Framework

The QOF was introduced as part of the nGMS.[9] In principle it is evidence based with indicators drawn from clinical and non-clinical areas, and with points attached to each, apparently according to their import and difficulty. For each point gained there is financial reward. This has a dual purpose, hence some of what you aspire to achieve is paid for in advance. Much of it needs to be invested in manpower resources if a practice is to have any hope of achieving high 'scores'. It also acts as a financial incentive to encourage the implementation and delivery of Evidence-Based Practice, and therefore has been a factor in increasing practice income. For many this is not the only incentive: the total number of points gained act as a personal incentive for some. Despite the lack of validity some local newspapers are already using these scores to create league tables. That the science behind this is weak has not stopped journalists publishing such data and regarding it as fact. This illustrates well another aspect of evaluating the quality of care that you deliver, that is, external evaluation. This could be a robust and valid assessment such as a Quality Practice Accreditation visit or a Primary Care Organisation sampling your QOF systems and achievement, but could be as crude as how you are represented in the local media. Like it or not, all are very real and in the new world of other companies being able to tender to provide medical services (Alternative Provider Medical Service providers) the quality of service you provide and how this is perceived and projected may be a key factor in determining your practice's future.

There are many respiratory QOF indicators, including for recording smoking status and for asthma and COPD. Those for asthma and COPD are shown in Table 13.2.

Table 13.2 ○ *The asthma and COPD Quality and Outcomes Framework indicators*

Asthma 1	The practice can produce a register of patients with asthma, excluding patients with asthma who have been prescribed no asthma-related drugs in the last 12 months
Asthma 8	The percentage of patients aged eight and over diagnosed as having asthma from 1 April 2006 with measures of variability or reversibility
Asthma 3	The percentage of patients with asthma between the ages of 14 and 19 in whom there is a record of smoking status in the previous 15 months
Asthma 6	The percentage of patients with asthma who have had an asthma review in the last 15 months
COPD 1	The practice can produce a register of patients with COPD
COPD 9	The percentage of all patients with COPD where diagnosis has been confirmed by spirometry including reversibility testing
COPD 10	The percentage of patients with COPD with a record of FEV_1 in the previous 15 months
COPD 11	The percentage of patients with COPD receiving inhaled treatment in whom there is a record that inhaler technique has been checked in the preceding 15 months
COPD 8	The percentage of patients with COPD who have had influenza immunisation in the preceding 1 September to 31 March

Note: the indicator numbers are no longer consecutive. When the QOF is revised and indicators removed those that replace them are given a new number to avoid confusion.

It is claimed that the QOF is evidence based and indeed this is true, as far as it can be. There is not a research secretariat testing all the evidence to produce the framework. The indicators were based on the best available evidence at the time, but often this was the best guidelines available at the time and, as we have already learned, these can be based on poor grades of evidence, even upon consensus only. This has led to areas of controversy. For example, one of the COPD indicators refers to spirometric reversibility testing for COPD. This was included based on the guidelines available at the time of the inception of nGMS but soon after its launch NICE issued new, more robust, guidelines questioning its reliability and laying down quite strict guidance. There is then a conflict that QOF encourages a test that NICE does not; you might consider this an ethical dilemma.

Self-evaluation

In the preceding sections we have largely focused on evaluating the quality of care provided by an organisation, typically a practice. Throughout there is the implicit suggestion that in so doing we would also be evaluating ourselves and our own practice. There has always been this expectation of independent professionals but gradually externally assured systems encroach on this professional responsibility and expect greater evidence of evaluation and reflection. The NHS appraisal system has been introduced with varying effect but it has at least encouraged personal reflection on our professional role. Examples of evidence that can be used for an appraisal also give us a useful indication of tools to help us self-evaluate. These include patient feedback, QOF scores, peer and staff feedback, prescribing data, referral data, personal elements of practice audit, thanks, compliments and sadly complaints, and not least personal significant events.

We will soon be required to participate in revalidation that will be divided into relicensing and recertification. Each UK doctor will require a licence to practise that will be renewed every five years, based upon annual appraisal but with a summative element. In addition recertification will be based upon fitness to continue in the doctor's chosen specialty, in our case general practice. This role has been foisted upon the medical royal colleges. The RCGP will now be walking a tightrope between delivering a robust recertification process and not been thought to be profiting from the process. The RCGP seeks to deliver this as a non-profit offering. There will no doubt be assessment tools but here GPs have a great strength. We are used to self-evaluation and used to providing evidence of this. This is an opportunity for GPs to develop their own acceptable yet valid means of demonstrating competence.

The majority of us now have robust systems in our practices, and sessional GPs collect a variety of information as they move around. We are in a strong position. Specialty registrars in the new GP specialty training programmes are in an even stronger position as they will be familiar with collecting evidence in order to gain the new MRCGP. It is important that as individuals we focus on professional performance rather than under-performance, that we reflect on our knowledge, skills and attitudes, and demonstrate our good practice. It will also be important to do this at an appropriate level. For example, a GP will need to demonstrate competence across the spectrum of primary care medicine; thus, the respiratory statement of the RCGP curriculum should give a good indicator of what is expected.[12] But if you aspire to be, or practise as, a GP with a Special Interest (GPwSI) in respiratory medicine you will not only need to be practising at a higher level but also be updating and demonstrating competence at this level.

Lifelong learning

Completing GP specialty training and gaining the MRCGP is but a step on a journey. The insightful GP will be daunted at the prospect of a lifetime of clinical practice and wondering how he or she will keep up to date. It is said that medical knowledge is doubling every 5 years and otherwise said that half of what we learn as fact at medical school will be disproven before we retire. Both may be urban myths but they are based on an underlying truth that medical knowledge is continually changing, and to keep up to date we need to be continually updating our knowledge and skills, and sometimes perhaps readjusting our attitudes. To stand still is to stagnate. But how do we determine in which areas to update, how do we do so and how can we demonstrate that we have done so? We cannot cover the whole of continuing professional development in this chapter, but a list of some useful resources is given below.

The field of respiratory medicine is changing rapidly. Research, not least pharmaceutical developments, is continually changing how we work. It is not too long ago that we were advised to tell our patients to 'double-up' their inhaled corticosteroids during an asthma exacerbation yet this is no longer advocated due to a paucity of evidence. You will need to consider how to keep up to date and how you identify learning needs. There are many possible approaches. Personal assessment relies on your ability to recognise knowledge and proficiency gaps on your insight and honesty. It is sensible to support this with external sources, feedback and with other assessments such as audits and appraisals. New guidelines and new QOF standards are in themselves often a trigger to learning. Many of us learned much more about spirometry after it was included in QOF and many updated their management of COPD following the launch of excellent new COPD guidelines from NICE. Other triggers such as the changes to oxygen prescription regulations gave an urgent need that many would not have previously seen as necessary. Some will see respiratory medicine as a personal interest, while for others it is just one of many areas in which a generalist needs to keep up to date. The balancing act of how and what to revisit, and how to adapt, is one that faces us throughout our professional lives. However, providing high-quality care and continually revisiting the care we give to ensure that we do so is part of the excitement and challenge that makes being a GP so rewarding.

Action points and learning points

▶ Consider how you evaluate medical evidence and how you share this evidence with a patient to enable him or her to make an informed treatment decision.
▶ Consider one of the following guidelines. What is their provenance? Are there any conflicts of interest? What grades of evidence are used to support the recommendations? Do you or would you use these guidelines in your normal clinical practice?
  ▷ BTS and SIGN • *British Guideline on the Management of Asthma.*
  ▷ BTS and SIGN • *British Guideline on the Management of Asthma in Children.*
  ▷ NICE • *Management of Chronic Obstructive Pulmonary Disease in Adults in Primary and Secondary Care.*
  ▷ Global Initiative for Chronic Obstructive Lung Disease • *Guide to COPD Diagnosis, Management and Prevention.*
▶ Having used this book, is there any area in which you would like to review the standard of care you provide? Consider the criteria and standards, and undertake an audit. Share the results with the primary healthcare team and consider what changes you would implement to improve the standard of care you offer.
▶ Imagine that the QOF criteria include an indicator that the latest guidelines suggest is no longer valid. Consider the ethical issues for yourself, the practice(s) in which you will be practising and for the other clinical staff that you might be asking to meet the needs of the QOF. You might like to consider that this indicator be based on a screening test and therefore apply criteria that evaluate screening tests (e.g. Singh–Wilson criteria). How will you handle this indicator in future?

▶ Consider your own professional practice. Are there areas of weakness that you wish to address? How can you demonstrate your strengths?

▶ How will you identify and address learning needs with regard to respiratory medicine throughout your career?

Further self–assessment

1 ▷ You might like to revisit your answers to the initial self-assessment. Would you amend any of your answers? Are you confident that spirometry is appropriately performed and interpreted in your current working environment?

2 ▷ You are a partner in a busy urban practice. You are the prescribing lead partner. A new asthma drug has been launched in an entirely new delivery device. The pharmaceutical company is promoting this heavily and making some astounding claims in the medical press and via their representatives. It has also supported, via an educational grant, a respiratory charity to advertise to patients in the lay press that asthma symptoms should be well controlled.

- How will you evaluate this new drug?
- How will you decide whether to use it yourself?
- What advice as prescribing lead will you give to other prescribers in your practice team?
- How will you manage enquiries from patients requesting the new 'asthma wonder drug'?
- What impact will this new drug have on the quality of care that you provide?
- How will you ascertain whether the quality of care you provide for your asthma patients is better in a year's time than it is now?

Further resources

Standards for Better Health • **www.dh.gov.uk/en/Publicationsand statistics/Publications/PublicationsPolicyAndGuidance/ DH_4086665** • this Department of Health document sets out a stand-ards framework for all NHS organisations and social service authorities.

RCGP Quality Practice Award (QPA) • **www.rcgp.org.uk/practising_ as_a_gp/team_quality/qpa.aspx** • this is a quality assurance proc-ess undertaken by practices, which recognises a high standard of quality patient care delivered by every member of the practice team. Each practice is required to submit a portfolio of written evidence set against 21 sets of criteria. This is set at a higher level than other quality initiatives.

Further reading

CLINICAL GOVERNANCE

van Zwanenberg T, Harrison J (eds). *Clinical Governance in Primary Care* (second edn), Abingdon: Radcliffe Publishing, 2004.

EVIDENCE-BASED PRACTICE

Gigerenzer G. *Reckoning with Risk: learning to live with uncertainty* London: Penguin, 2002.

Muir Gray JA. *Evidence-Based Healthcare: how to make health policy and management decisions* London: Churchill Livingstone, 2001.

Risdale L. *Evidence-Based General Practice: a critical reader* London: WB Saunders 1995.

Guidelines – compendium published by Medendium • **www.eguidelines.co.uk**.

AUDIT

National Institute for Health and Clinical Excellence. *Principles for Best Practice in Clinical Audit* Abingdon: Radcliffe Publishing, 2002.

SIGNIFICANT EVENT REVIEW

Royal College of General Practitioners. *Significant Event Auditing* (Occasional Paper 70) London: RCGP, 1995.

LIFELONG LEARNING

Pietroni R. *The Toolbox for Portfolio Development* Abingdon: Radcliffe Publishing, 2001.
Rughani A. *The GP's Guide to Personal Development Plans* Abingdon: Radcliffe Publishing, 2000.

Wakely G, Chambers R, Field S. *Continuing Professional Development in Primary Care: making it happen* Abingdon: Radcliffe Publishing, 2000.

References

1 • Bolam v Friern Hospital Management Committee (1957) 1 WLR 583.

2 • Department of Health. *The New NHS: modern, dependable* London: The Stationery Office, 1997.

3 • Rawlinson M. Foreword. In: T van Zwanenberg, J Harrison (eds). *Clinical Governance in Primary Care* Abingdon: Radcliffe Publishing, 2000.

4 • van Zwanenberg T, Edwards C. Clinical governance in primary care, in T van Zwanenberg, J Harrison (eds). *Clinical Governance in Primary Care* Abingdon: Radcliffe Publishing, 2000, pp. 18–19.

5 • Department of Health. *Standards for Better Health* London: The Stationery Office, 2006.

6 • Sackett D L, Rosenberg W M C, Gray J A M, *et al.* Evidence based medicine: what it is and what it isn't *British Medical Journal* 1996; **312**: 71–2.

7 • Gigerenzer G. *Reckoning with Risk* London: Penguin, 2002.

8 • Scott R. *Report of the Inquiry into the Export of Defence Equipment and Dual-Use Goods to Iraq and Related Prosecutions* London: HMSO, 1996.

9 • British Medical Association and NHS Confederation. *New GMS Contract 2003 Investing in General Practice: supporting documentation* London: BMA and NHS Confederation, 2003.

10 • National Institute for Health and Clinical Excellence. *Principles for Best Practice in Clinical Audit* Abingdon: Radcliffe Publishing, 2002.

11 • Royal College of General Practitioners. *Significant Event Auditing* (Occasional Paper 70) London: RCGP, 1995.

12 • Royal College of General Practitioners. *Respiratory Problems* (Curriculum Statement 15.8) London: RCGP, 2007, www.rcgp-curriculum.org.uk/PDF/curr_15_8_Respiratory_problems.pdf [accessed January 2009].

263

Appendix: resources

Monica Fletcher and Simon Gregory

There are disease area-specific resources listed throughout this book. The aim of this chapter is to provide quick access to resources should you wish to look into respiratory medicine in greater depth. Realistically the bulk of these are now most easily accessed on the internet. The editors and the RCGP are not responsible for the content of these sites. If any of the links listed are broken they can usually be found via any popular search engine.

General respiratory education, resources and support

Education for Health • **www.educationforhealth.org.uk** • offers a range of courses and educational resources including books, visual aids and patient materials.

The *General Practice Airways Group* • **www.gpiag.org** • is a primary care-based organisation that provides a variety or resources, including the *Primary Care Respiratory Journal* and a website with a useful list of links to other sites. This links page includes the majority of sites and resources that are relevant to respiratory medicine. Since sites are dynamic they are not all listed here.

Guidelines

National Institute for Health and Clinical Excellence (NICE) • **www.nice.org.uk** • has a plethora of clinical guidelines. The following are pertinent:
▷ *Clinical Guideline 12, Chronic Obstructive Pulmonary Disease*
▷ *Clinical Guideline 24, Lung Cancer*
▷ *Clinical Guideline 33, Tuberculosis.*

Scottish Intercollegiate Guidelines Network (SIGN) • **www.sign.ac.uk** • has a robust cross-inclusive approach that has produced a wide range of excellent guidelines, including:

▷ **SIGN 59** • *Community Management of Lower Respiratory Tract Infection in Adults*

▷ **SIGN 63** • *British Guideline on the Management of Asthma*

▷ **SIGN 73** • *Management of Obstructive Sleep Apnoea/Hypopnoea in Adults*

▷ **SIGN 80** • *Management of Patients with Lung Cancer*

▷ **SIGN 91** • *Bronchiolitis in Children*.

The *British Thoracic Society* (BTS) • **www.brit-thoracic.org.uk** • has an excellent site with many resources including audit tools and guidelines. The clinical information section is a rich area.

The *Global Initiative for Chronic Obstructive Lung Disease* (GOLD) • **www.goldcopd.com** • has international COPD guidelines and resources.

The *Global Initiative for Asthma* (GINA) • **www.ginasthma.com** • has similar resources and guidelines pertaining to asthma.

Further information sources

The Lung and Asthma Information Agency (LAIA) • **www.laia.ac.uk**.

Respiratory NHS Electronic Library • **www.library.nhs.uk/ RESPIRATORY**.

Clinical support

Spirometry

SpirXpert • **www.spirxpert.com** • is an excellent site for information about this tricky area, including training materials and software to aid interpretation.

Smoking cessation

The *International Primary Care Respiratory Group* smoking support pages • **www.theipcrg.org** • are good, simple resources for the busy GP.

Journals

Primary Care Respiratory Journal • **www.thepcrj.org**.

Thorax • **www.thorax.bmj.com**.

British Journal of General Practice • **www.rcgp.org.uk/bjgp**.

The Lancet • **www.thelancet.com**.

New England Journal of Medicine • **www.nejm.org**.

British Medical Journal • **www.bmj.com**.

Patient organisations

The Anaphylaxis Campaign • **www.anaphylaxis.org.uk**.

Asthma UK • **www.asthma.org.uk**.

Allergy UK • **www.allergyuk.org**.

British Lung Foundation • **www.lunguk.org**.

Cancerbackup (was BACUP) • **www.cancerbackup.org.uk**.

Cystic Fibrosis Trust • **www.cftrust.org.uk**.

Index

271

277